Your Pregnancy
WEEK *by* WEEK

Your Pregnancy

WEEK *by* WEEK

ALISON MACKONOCHIE

A VERY SPECIAL THANK YOU TO ROBIN FOR HIS UNFAILING SUPPORT, TO LUCY AND KATE, WITHOUT WHOM
WE WOULD NOT HAVE HAD CHRISTMAS, AND TO DOMINIC FOR JUST BEING HIMSELF.

This edition published by Smithmark Publishers,
a division of U.S. Media Holdings, Inc.
16 East 32nd Street, New York, NY 10016

SMITHMARK books are available for bulk purchase for sales
promotion and premium use. For details write or call the manager of
special sales, SMITHMARK Publishers, 16 East 32nd Street,
New York, NY 10016; (212) 532-6600

© Anness Publishing Limited 1996

This book was previously published as part of a larger compendium,
The Complete Book of Pregnancy & Babycare.

Produced by
Anness Publishing Limited
1 Boundary Row
London SE1 8HP

ISBN 0-8317-7221-2

Publisher: Joanna Lorenz
Project Editors: Casey Horton, Nicky Thompson
Editor: Elizabeth Longley
Designer: Bobbie Colgate Stone
Jacket Designer: Patrick Mcleavey & Partners
Special Photography: Alistair Hughes
Additional Photography: Carin Simon
Illustrations: Ian Sidaway
Hair and Make-up: Bettina Graham

Printed in Singapore by Star Standard Industries Pte. Ltd.

ACKNOWLEDGMENTS

The author and publisher would like to thank the many individuals
who helped in the creation of this book. In particular thanks are due
to Bobbie Brown, Elsa Jacobi, Pauline Richardson, Mary Lambert and
Jane Barret. Many thanks also go to everyone who modelled for special
photography: Yvonne Adams and Martin; Ruth Auber and Bethany;
Jo Bates and Lois; Amanda Bennet-Jones; Kim, Neil and Andrew
Brown; Christine Clarke; Jacqueline Clarke and Cassia; Jocelyn
Cusack and Beth; Sam Dyas and Colt; Patricia Gannon and Matthew;
Nici Giles and Fergus; Yiota Gillis and Cameron; Sandra Hadfield and
Annie; Louise Henriques and Joshua; Lynette Jones and Hugh and
Rhys; Karen, Mark, Megan and Robert Lambert; Claire Lehain and
Harriet; Lavinia Mainds and Polly; Pippa Milton and Oliver; Philippa
Madden and Inca; Jackie Norbury; Jess Presland; Katey Steiner;
Saatchi Spracklen and Niamh; Sophie Trotter and Archie; Josephine
Whitfield and Lily May; Lucinda Whitrow and Hector. Thanks also to
companies who loaned items and photographs: Blooming Marvellous
Ltd (pages 36-37), Boots Children's Wear and Toys, Fisher-Price,
Littlewoods Home Shopping, Maclaren Ltd and Mattel UK Ltd.

Picture acknowledgments: **Bubbles** 74; /Jacquie Farrow, 64; /Julie
Fisher 5, /Nikki Gibbs 12 b, 76, /Paul Howard 71 t, /Julia Martin 17
b, 81 (all 3); /Loisjoy Thurston 1, 25 b, 43 t and r 48, 60, 77; /Ian
West 73 b; /J. Woodcock 25 t, 74; /Richard Yard 65; **Lupe Cunha**
14, 15, 17 t and b, 19, 22, 23 b, 29 t and b, 35 t, 48, 49 t, 57 bl and t,
57 r, 69 t, 78, 79 r and tr, 82, 83; **PR Communications** 50 (box);
Science Photo Library/BSIP Bajande 85 b; /Mark Clarke 56, 57 t,
68, 69 b, 70, 71 b, 75 r, 84 t and b, 85 t and b; /Custom Medical
Stock 57 t, 85 t; /Simon Fraser 43, 69 b; /Will & Deni McIntyre 20 t,
21 b; /Joseph Mettis 68; /Petit Format/Nestle 12 t; /Chris Priest 32;
35; /Richard G Rawlins 11 tl, 20 t, 21 b, 31, 32; /Pascale Roche/
Petit Format 84 t and b; /James Stevenson 16 br, 31 b, 43 bl; /Ron
Sutherland 75 r; /Sheila Terry 17 t, 61, 79 bl; /Jonathan Watts 56;
Carin Simon 76 r.
(**Key**: b – bottom, bl – bottom left, br – bottom right, r – right, t –
top, tl – top left, tr – top right).
The publishers have tried to credit all agencies and photographers
whose pictures appear in this book and apologize for any omissions.

CONTENTS

INTRODUCTION

PREGNANCY IS A VERY SPECIAL TIME for both you and your partner. Knowing what is happening to you and your growing baby during the weeks ahead will help you both to enjoy this exciting period in your lives. Starting with pre-pregnancy care, this book explains how conception takes place and then looks at pregnancy and your baby's development week by week. Many of the issues raised will be relevant throughout your pregnancy and not just during the week in which they are first mentioned, so do read it all.

It is normal to experience some minor discomforts during pregnancy and you will want to know how to cope with them. More serious problems can occasionally occur, and it is important to recognize the symptoms so that you will know when immediate medical treatment is required. The birth is something you may feel anxious about and it will help you if you understand the choices available in both prenatal care and childbirth. By being informed you will be able to choose the type of care and birth that is right for you.

As your body adapts to the changes that pregnancy brings, you will begin to prepare yourself physically, emotionally and practically for parenthood. A well-balanced, healthy diet is essential for both your well-being and that of your baby. Exercise has an important part to play too, not just in keeping you fit but also in preparing your body for the birth. Looking good will help you to feel good, so you should take special care of your physical appearance throughout your pregnancy. Knowing how to select the right clothes to suit your changing shape and how to use makeup to emphasize your best features will help you to feel confident and make your pregnancy an even more enjoyable experience.

PREPARING FOR PREGNANCY

Once you have decided that you want to have a baby, you and your partner should concentrate on getting yourselves fit and healthy before you try to conceive. Ideally, you should begin preparing for pregnancy at least three months before conception so that you can be sure that your child will get the best possible start in life. If your pregnancy is unplanned, then start taking extra care of yourself as soon as you suspect that you might be pregnant. This may involve some basic changes in your lifestyle.

There is evidence that suggests that smoking by either partner can delay conception, so if you or your partner smoke you should stop now. In addition, smoking during pregnancy will put the baby at risk and can also affect your well-being; giving up before conception will benefit you and your child.

Alcohol can inhibit fertility, so both you and your partner should avoid drinking alcohol while trying to conceive. Once you are pregnant alcohol can restrict fetal development and could even cause malformation. Since there is no safe limit for alcohol during pregnancy it is better to give it up altogether.

MEDICATION

Fertilization and the early development of a baby are controlled by delicately balanced chemical processes in the body. Additional chemicals entering your body as medication can upset this development, so if possible you should avoid taking any medicines before conception and during pregnancy. If you are on long-term medication, you will need to talk to your doctor about your options. Medicines that are available over the counter, natural remedies and vitamin supplements should also be avoided, unless they have been recommended by your doctor.

Oral contraceptives rely on chemically-produced hormones to control fertility. If you are taking the pill, change to a barrier method, such as the condom or diaphragm, for three months before trying to conceive. This allows your body to clear itself of synthetic hormones and to re-establish its own cycle.

IMMUNIZATIONS

An unborn baby exposed to rubella (German measles) during its early development can be born severely handicapped. Don't assume that because you were vaccinated in your teens, or you have had the infection, that you are automatically immune. Ask your doctor to give you a blood

Before trying for a baby, both partners should get fit by walking and other exercise.

Salmon is ideal as part of a balanced diet, because it is low in fat but full of vitamins.

By doing regular stretching exercises at home, or at an organized class, you will strengthen yourself for pregnancy.

As your legs have to carry more weight during pregnancy, try to do regular daily exercises such as running in place to build them up.

test to check. If you are not immune you can be vaccinated, but you should not get pregnant until the vaccine virus has cleared from your blood, which takes about three months. If you have been given vaccines for tropical diseases, you should also wait for three months before getting pregnant.

NUTRITION AND EXERCISE

A well-balanced, healthy diet that contains reasonable daily amounts of carbohydrate, protein, fat, minerals, and vitamins is essential for both your well-being and that of your baby. Everything you eat will also become your unborn child's nourishment, and what you store before pregnancy is important for early fetal development when all the major organs are formed.

One of the B vitamins, folic acid, helps prevent neural tube defects (NTD), such as spina bifida, in unborn babies. It is recommended that all women planning a pregnancy should increase their average daily intake to 0.6 mg by taking a 0.4 mg supplement before attempting conception, and during the first 12 weeks of pregnancy. This is the time when your baby's organs and body systems are forming.

Regular exercise, such as brisk walking or swimming, is important if you are to maintain a healthy lifestyle. Exercise will help you get fit before conception and, as your pregnancy progresses, it will strengthen muscles in your lower back, stomach, and legs, which will help your body cope better with the demands of pregnancy.

THE FIRST TRIMESTER

WEEKS 1–4: CONCEPTION

During the first half of the menstrual cycle two chemical substances called hormones are released from special glands into the bloodstream. One hormone stimulates the process that results in the production of an ovum, or ripe egg. The other hormone stimulates the endometrium, or lining of the uterus (womb), to thicken in readiness to receive a fertilized ovum. About two weeks from the end of your menstrual cycle the work of the first hormone is completed and you ovulate; that is, a ripe ovum is released from one of your ovaries. Conception occurs if your partner's sperm fertilizes this ovum. This usually takes place in the fallopian tube that connects the ovary to the uterus. The fertilized ovum completes its journey to the uterus, where it implants into the thickened uterine lining. Once this process occurs the cervix increases slightly in width and becomes softer, and a thick mucous plug seals off the uterus to protect it from infection. After two weeks, if there has been no conception, the thickened uterine lining is shed and menstruation takes place.

AFTER FERTILIZATION

The fertilized single-cell egg multiplies into two, then four cells, and it continues multiplying so that by about day seven, when it reaches the uterus, it has grown into a ball of over 100 cells with a fluid-filled cavity. This ball, called a blastocyst, has two layers: the outer one becomes the placenta, while the inner one forms the embryo, which develops into your baby.

The embryo is made up of three layers of tissue, each of which forms separately. The outer layer develops into the nerves and skin; the middle layer forms the bones, cartilage, muscles, circulatory system, kidneys, and sex organs; and the inner layer

You and your body

You won't be aware of the changes that are happening inside your body during these early weeks, although it is possible that you may experience very slight bleeding at the time when your next period would have been due. Usually the first indication that you are pregnant will be a missed period.

becomes the respiratory and digestive systems.

The placenta is the unborn baby's life-support system. It is attached to the lining of the uterus and separates the developing baby's circulation

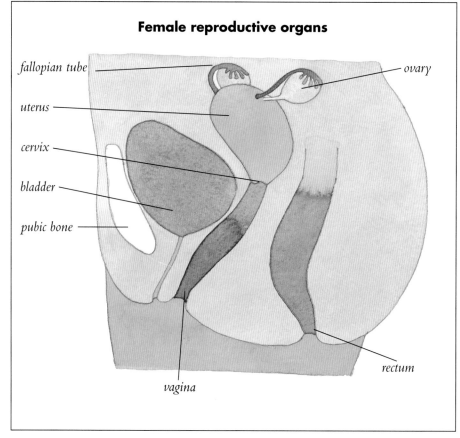

Female reproductive organs

fallopian tube — ovary
uterus —
cervix —
bladder —
pubic bone —
rectum
vagina

If an egg in the fallopian tube is fertilized by a sperm, it will embed itself into the lining of the uterus. If not, it is shed down through the cervix and out through the vagina.

This fertilized egg now has two cells called blastomeres and is the primitive embryo. It will multiply to over 100 cells.

An enlarged sperm and ovum

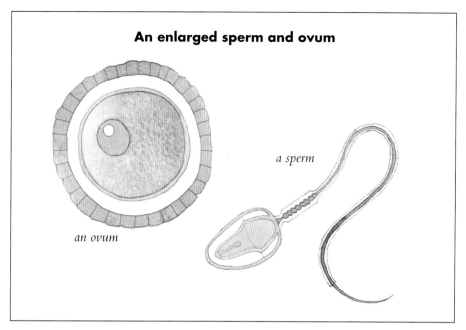

a sperm

an ovum

A sperm and an ovum are tiny. A man ejaculates about 500 million sperm, while a woman usually produces one ovum half-way through her menstrual cycle.

from its mother's. It allows oxygen and food, as well as protective antibodies, to pass from the mother along the umbilical cord to the baby. The placenta isn't fully formed until the end of the 12th week of pregnancy when it is able to take over the production of the pregnancy

hormones estrogen and progesterone, from the ovaries.

Within the uterus, the embryo is contained in the amniotic sac. This

is filled with fluid in which the developing child will float until birth. The amniotic fluid offers protection from any external pressures.

THE BABY'S SEX

A child's sex is determined by the father's sperm at the time of conception. Sperm carry either an X or Y chromosome while the egg has only an X chromosome. If a Y-chromosome sperm fertilizes the egg, the baby will be a boy. If the sperm carries an X chromosome, the baby will be a girl.

Male reproductive organs

bladder

seminal vesicle

vas deferens

penis

foreskin

glans

scrotum   testis

rectum

Sperm mature in both testes. When a man is sexually aroused, the penis becomes erect and the outlet from the bladder into the ejaculatory duct is closed leaving it free for sperm.

Trimesters

Pregnancy lasts approximately 40 weeks and is calculated from the first day of your last period, although conception will probably not have taken place until around two weeks after this. Pregnancy is divided into three parts known as trimesters. The first covers weeks 1–13, the second trimester weeks 14–26, and the third trimester week 27 until birth.

WEEK 5: CONFIRMING PREGNANCY

Pregnancy can be confirmed by means of a simple test that measures the levels of the pregnancy hormone human chorionic gonadotrophin (HCG) that are present in your urine. The test can be carried out as soon as you reach the day that your next period should have started. Your doctor or family planning clinic will do the test, or you may prefer to perform a home test yourself using one of the kits available from the pharmacist. Ensure that you choose a kit that will give an accurate result this early. Although many modern home-testing kits state that you can test your urine at any time, you may wish to use an early morning sample because this urine will contain the highest concentration of HCG.

If the result is positive, you must make an appointment to see your doctor so that he or she can make

Your growing baby

Although the embryo is only just visible to the naked eye, the spinal column and brain have already begun to grow and a blood vessel has developed which will become the heart. The embryo is ⅛ in long.

arrangements for your prenatal care and the birth.

EARLY SYMPTOMS
Some women experience all the early symptoms of pregnancy, while others sail through the first weeks without any feelings of discomfort.
• Your body is having to work hard to adapt to the demands of pregnancy, so you may feel overwhelmingly tired. Try to get as much rest as possible. You will find that sitting with your feet up for even half an hour will help.
• Your breasts may tingle or feel tender, rather as they do before a period; your nipples will appear darker and more prominent and the veins will be more noticeable. You should wear a good support bra from now until after your baby is born.
• You may experience a strange metallic taste in the mouth, which

If you're lucky, you'll experience no nausea in pregnancy and continue exercising as normal.

You and your body

This is the first week that you will be able to confirm that you are pregnant.

To confirm a pregnancy, you can do a test with a kit from a pharmacist, but ensure you choose one that is suitable to use for a test at five weeks.

During the day try eating six high-carbohydrate meals, such as pasta, potato, and bread. Avoid rich or fatty foods.

• Finally, as the enlarging uterus presses on your bladder you may need to urinate more frequently.

DATING THE BIRTH

Once your pregnancy is confirmed, you will want to know your baby's likely date of birth. You can calculate an estimated date of delivery (EDD) by counting 40 weeks from the first day of your last period. But you should remember that since you don't know the exact date of ovulation this EDD is approximate. At about 10 weeks the fetal heartbeat can be measured with a Doppler device.

can be accompanied by an aversion to certain foods and tea and coffee.

• A feeling of nausea, or even actual vomiting in the morning or at any time during the day, is quite usual. It is often worse when your stomach is empty, so have a few light crackers before you get up in the morning.

Estimated date of delivery

JANUARY	1 2 3 4 5 6 7 8 9 10 11 12 13 14 15 16 17 18 19 20 21 22 23 24 25 26 27 28 29 30 31	JANUARY
OCTOBER	8 9 10 11 12 13 14 15 16 17 18 19 20 21 22 23 24 25 26 27 28 29 30 31 1 2 3 4 5 6 7	NOVEMBER
FEBRUARY	1 2 3 4 5 6 7 8 9 10 11 12 13 14 15 16 17 18 19 20 21 22 23 24 25 26 27 28	FEBRUARY
NOVEMBER	8 9 10 11 12 13 14 15 16 17 18 19 20 21 22 23 24 25 26 27 28 29 30 1 2 3 4 5	DECEMBER
MARCH	1 2 3 4 5 6 7 8 9 10 11 12 13 14 15 16 17 18 19 20 21 22 23 24 25 26 27 28 29 30 31	MARCH
DECEMBER	6 7 8 9 10 11 12 13 14 15 16 17 18 19 20 21 22 23 24 25 26 27 28 29 30 31 1 2 3 4 5	JANUARY
APRIL	1 2 3 4 5 6 7 8 9 10 11 12 13 14 15 16 17 18 19 20 21 22 23 24 25 26 27 28 29 30	APRIL
JANUARY	6 7 8 9 10 11 12 13 14 15 16 17 18 19 20 21 22 23 24 25 26 27 28 29 30 31 1 2 3 4	FEBRUARY
MAY	1 2 3 4 5 6 7 8 9 10 11 12 13 14 15 16 17 18 19 20 21 22 23 24 25 26 27 28 29 30 31	MAY
FEBRUARY	5 6 7 8 9 10 11 12 13 14 15 16 17 18 19 20 21 22 23 24 25 26 27 28 1 2 3 4 5 6 7	MARCH
JUNE	1 2 3 4 5 6 7 8 9 10 11 12 13 14 15 16 17 18 19 20 21 22 23 24 25 26 27 28 29 30	JUNE
MARCH	8 9 10 11 12 13 14 15 16 17 18 19 20 21 22 23 24 25 26 27 28 29 30 31 1 2 3 4 5 6	APRIL
JULY	1 2 3 4 5 6 7 8 9 10 11 12 13 14 15 16 17 18 19 20 21 22 23 24 25 26 27 28 29 30 31	JULY
APRIL	7 8 9 10 11 12 13 14 15 16 17 18 19 20 21 22 23 24 25 26 27 28 29 30 1 2 3 4 5 6 7	MAY
AUGUST	1 2 3 4 5 6 7 8 9 10 11 12 13 14 15 16 17 18 19 20 21 22 23 24 25 26 27 28 29 30 31	AUGUST
MAY	8 9 10 11 12 13 14 15 16 17 18 19 20 21 22 23 24 25 26 27 28 29 30 31 1 2 3 4 5 6 7	JUNE
SEPTEMBER	1 2 3 4 5 6 7 8 9 10 11 12 13 14 15 16 17 18 19 20 21 22 23 24 25 26 27 28 29 30	SEPTEMBER
JUNE	8 9 10 11 12 13 14 15 16 17 18 19 20 21 22 23 24 25 26 27 28 29 30 1 2 3 4 5 6 7	JULY
OCTOBER	1 2 3 4 5 6 7 8 9 10 11 12 13 14 15 16 17 18 19 20 21 22 23 24 25 26 27 28 29 30 31	OCTOBER
JULY	8 9 10 11 12 13 14 15 16 17 18 19 20 21 22 23 24 25 26 27 28 29 30 31 1 2 3 4 5 6 7	AUGUST
NOVEMBER	1 2 3 4 5 6 7 8 9 10 11 12 13 14 15 16 17 18 19 20 21 22 23 24 25 26 27 28 29 30	NOVEMBER
AUGUST	8 9 10 11 12 13 14 15 16 17 18 19 20 21 22 23 24 25 26 27 28 29 30 31 1 2 3 4 5 6	SEPTEMBER
DECEMBER	1 2 3 4 5 6 7 8 9 10 11 12 13 14 15 16 17 18 19 20 21 22 23 24 25 26 27 28 29 30 31	DECEMBER
SEPTEMBER	7 8 9 10 11 12 13 14 15 16 17 18 19 20 21 22 23 24 25 26 27 28 29 30 1 2 3 4 5 6 7	OCTOBER

Find the first day of your last period on the white bands; the date on the tint band below is your EDD.

WEEK 6: PRENATAL CHOICES

If you haven't already, now is the time to select a practitioner to care for you before and during the birth. In the U.S., most babies are still delivered in a hospital by an obstetrician-gynecologist, though many women are increasingly opting for the services of a certified nurse-midwife. Another choice is the maternity center, which is staffed with nurse-midwives and has one or more physicians on call in case difficulties arise. If you choose to have a midwife assist with the birth, you may still want to see an obstetrician-gynecologist for part or all of your prenatal care.

Women choose a midwife over an OB-GYN for a number of reasons, but two of the most common are the desire for a more natural, less medicalized birth, and the feeling that midwives offer greater sympathy for both physical and emotional issues than most physicians. Before making any decisions, of course, you should consult your health insurance plan to determine which services are covered, and to what extent.

If you have reason to believe that yours may be a high-risk pregnancy, you may want to consider yet another option – a high-risk specialist. Factors that could lead to a pregnancy

being classified as high-risk include certain chronic medical conditions (such as diabetes or lupus), previous pregnancy losses, or advanced maternal age (though more and more older women are having healthy, normal pregnancies). A high-risk specialist, also known as a perinatalogist or maternal-fetal specialist, can act as a consultant to your own

You and your body

If you are suffering from morning sickness, you may find that the smell of certain things, such as tobacco smoke or frying food, brings on the sickness or makes it worse. The texture of your skin may become dry and flaky, or you may break out. Now is the time to start thinking about your prenatal care, and the type of birth you want.

In a home birth, a midwife will often palpate your abdomen, to feel the top of the uterus (fundus).

doctor or alternatively function as your primary caregiver.

If for any reason your pregnancy becomes "high-risk" as it progresses, you can bring in a specialist at any stage. One advantage to being treated by this kind of practitioner is that it offers the anxious mother increased interaction with her doctor and an enhanced sense of control over her pregnancy. It's helpful, too, to remember that most so-called high-risk pregnancies result in the birth of healthy babies.

The actual care you get will be similar wherever you receive it, because all prenatal care is designed to ensure that you and your unborn baby remain healthy during pregnancy.

These days, the best pattern of prenatal care for a healthy woman is considered to be no more than nine prenatal appointments. If you have any concerns between these appointments, you can telephone your doctor or midwife for advice.

HOME BIRTH

A home birth means you give birth in the familiar surroundings of your own home under the supervision of a midwife. If you want to deliver your baby in this way, you will need to talk to your doctor to see whether there are any medical reasons why this isn't advisable. Home births, though relatively common in Europe and Great Britain, are still extremely rare in this country.

HOSPITAL BIRTH

Most women still prefer a hospital birth because they feel safer knowing that there will be experts on hand to help if there are any complications. Also, if the baby needs special care this will be available almost immediately. Although hospitals are no

You will usually spend between two to three days in the hospital when you give birth, depending on your delivery.

longer the dictatorial places they used to be, and most try to cater to parents' wishes, not all of them are able to offer every type of birth. You will need to find out what facilities your hospital offers. Often your doctor will be affiliated with a certain hospital and will direct you there. Most hospitals offer childbirth education classes which include a tour of the labor and birthing rooms and the nursery. It is very important to check your insurance plan as there are varying types of coverage for semi-private and private rooms, anaesthesia and length of stay. Many insurance companies allow only one overnight hospital stay for a vaginal delivery with no complications, but offer follow-up home care. Before

making your decision talk to other mothers who have had their babies there recently.

Your growing baby

The heart has now formed in the chest cavity and is beginning to beat. By the end of this week the stalk connecting the embryo to the placenta will have begun to grow into the umbilical cord and blood vessels will have started to form. The embryo is now about the size of your little fingernail and its movements can be picked up by ultrasound scan. The head has the beginning of the eyes, ears, and mouth and there are tiny buds which will become arms and legs.

WEEK 7: POSSIBLE PROBLEMS

Although the majority of pregnancies go without a hitch, sometimes serious problems do occur and special care is needed. Complications can usually be resolved with monitoring, but occasionally the pregnancy comes to an end. Although the following conditions are not likely to affect you, you should be aware of their symptoms:

Preeclampsia (pregnancy-induced hypertension) This is a high blood pressure condition that is sometimes associated with a reduction in the quality of placental function. If preeclampsia is left untreated it can cut the oxygen flow to the fetus and put it at risk; the fetal growth rate may also be affected. Symptoms include elevated blood pressure, protein in the urine and, occasionally, headache. You will be tested for signs of preeclampsia at each prenatal visit. In the early stages preeclampsia may be treated with complete bedrest or medication under medical supervision. Later in the pregnancy, if the condition is severe, it may become necessary to induce the birth. The mother's blood pressure will soon return to normal. If the condition is left completely untreated it can develop into eclampsia, which can be fatal for both the mother and the child. Today, this condition is extremely rare, and most cases don't occur until at least the twentieth week.

Bleeding in early pregnancy

Bleeding or spotting from the vagina is known as a threatened miscarriage. It is possible to bleed quite heavily and not miscarry or do any harm to the baby. All bleeding in pregnancy must be taken seriously, however, and you should report it to your doctor immediately. Your doctor is likely to carry out an internal pelvic examination and arrange for you to have an ultrasound scan to see whether the baby is developing normally. Providing everything is all right you will probably be told to rest until the bleeding stops.

Ectopic pregnancy This occurs when the fertilized egg implants itself in one of the fallopian tubes rather than in the uterus. If it is undetected, the growing baby even-

You and your body

You may feel dizzy or even faint if you stand for too long or you are in a crowd. Overwhelming exhaustion can also be a problem now, so make sure you get plenty of rest. If you don't feel like making love at the moment don't worry; this is quite normal and you may find that your sex life is better then ever in the second trimester.

Your growing baby

The unborn baby is now known as a fetus and is about ½ in long. The nostrils, lips, tongue, and teeth are beginning to form and the arms and legs are growing. The lungs are beginning to develop and the intestines, spine, and the brain are now almost fully developed.

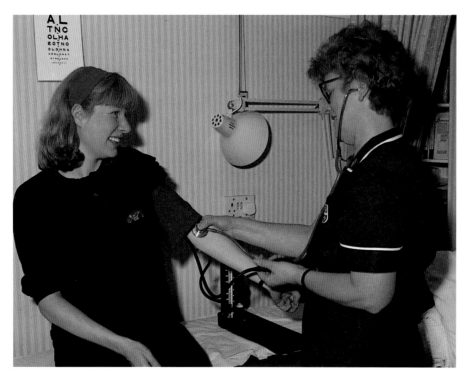

Regular blood pressure checks are essential at prenatal visits to detect preeclampsia.

tually ruptures the tube, which causes severe pain. Immediate surgery is required to terminate the pregnancy, and this often means losing the fallopian tube as well. In extreme cases the ovary may also have to be removed. If the other ovary and fallopian tube are healthy, there is no reason why another successful pregnancy should not take place.

If the ectopic pregnancy is discovered early enough, a drug can be given that causes the embryo to be reabsorbed by the body; this prevents the fallopian tube from bursting. Symptoms of an ectopic pregnancy include pain in the side of the abdomen, vaginal bleeding, and fainting.

Miscarriage The most common time for miscarriage is during the first three months of pregnancy, although losing a baby at any time before the 24th week is described as a miscarriage. Some miscarriages occur for no known reason. Known causes of miscarriage include hormonal problems, disease or infection,

You will have a number of blood tests throughout your pregnancy but these are no cause for alarm. The tests are simply a means for your doctor to make sure that you are progressing normally and not experiencing any problems.

abnormalities of the uterus, or an incompetent cervix. If this last condition is known to exist, it can be dealt with by a surgical suture that will be removed before the EDD.

Although it is unlikely that sexual intercourse will cause miscarriage,

women who have experienced bleeding early in their pregnancy or who are known to have a tendency to miscarry are usually advised by doctors not to have intercourse for the first 12 weeks, until their pregnancy is well established.

You may start to feel very tired in these early weeks, so get plenty of rest and make sure your feet are propped up.

WEEK 8: ROUTINE TESTS

Your first prenatal check-up will usually take place between eight and 12 weeks, and will almost certainly be the most thorough of all your prenatal visits. You will be asked a lot of personal questions about your health, family medical history, and possibly even about your and your partner's jobs and living accommodations. All this information is required to build up a picture of you and your pregnancy so that any potential risks can be spotted and help can be offered where it is particularly needed.

If you have any questions or worries about your pregnancy, this is a good time to discuss them. It's easy to forget to ask something important when there is so much to take in at one time, so it may be helpful to write down a list of things that you want to know about before you attend the exam.

ROUTINE TESTS

Certain tests are carried out during pregnancy to ensure that both you and the fetus are progressing well. Some of these will be repeated at each prenatal visit; others will only be carried out at the initial exam.

Blood pressure This will be taken at each visit. Increased blood pressure could develop into preeclampsia, which could endanger both you and the fetus.

Urine You will be asked to give a sample of urine at each prenatal visit. This will be tested for any infections that may require some treatment, as well as for sugar, protein, or the chemical substances known as ketones. Sugar in the urine could be a sign of diabetes; protein may indicate the onset of preeclampsia; and ketones may indicate that your kidneys are being adversely affected by your progressing pregnancy.

You and your body

The changes to your body are becoming more noticeable as your breasts and nipples enlarge and become sensitive. Your vagina changes from light to dark pink, and you may notice an increased vaginal discharge.

It is time for regular monitoring of your pregnancy.

Weight Your weight will almost certainly be monitored regularly to see how the baby is growing. You can expect to gain anything from 20 lb to 40 lb during your pregnancy, with most of this extra weight going on after the 20th week. A sudden increase in weight could be an indication of preeclampsia.

Height You will be measured at your first appointment because your height gives a rough guide to

---

Weight gain during pregnancy

Baby 39%

Blood 22%

Amniotic fluid 11%

Uterus 11%

Placenta 9%

Breasts 8%

Your weight increases by about 1–2 lb weekly during months four to eight, with very little in the last month. As your breasts get larger, the uterus, placenta and baby develop, and the amniotic fluid increases, until they reach the percentages shown here.

The amount of weight that you will gain during pregnancy varies, depending on your height and size, but can be as much as 40 lb.

At your first prenatal check-up, a blood sample will be taken to find out your blood group and type, and to make sure you're not anemic or carrying a virus such as hepatitis B. You will have blood tests regularly through your pregnancy.

you are of Afro-American descent, they will probably test for sickle-cell disease. Blood-testing for the HIV or AIDS virus is not routinely done at hospitals, except by special request of the mother.

Internal examination You may have an internal examination at your first visit. This is to check for any abnormalities of the vagina, cervix, or the uterus. If you haven't had a cervical Pap smear during the last three to five years you may well be given one.

Wrists and ankles These will be checked at each visit for any noticeable swelling, or edema, caused by fluid retention, since these signs could possibly indicate that the mother has preeclampsia.

Palpation The doctor or midwife will palpate, that is press, your abdomen to feel the top of the uterus (fundus). He or she will then feel down toward the pelvis to check the size of the fetus and the way it is lying in the uterus.

Your growing baby

The fetus is now about 1 in long, which is 10,000 times bigger than at conception. All the major organs are present, although still developing. The ears and eyes have formed and the skin covering the eyes will eventually split to form the eyelids. The middle ear, which controls balance as well as hearing, is also developing. The heart is now pumping with a regular beat, and blood vessels can be seen. As the arms and legs grow longer, the fetus begins to move around and starts to kick, although it is still too small at this stage for you to be able to feel it or detect any movement.

the size of your pelvis. If your pelvis is too small to accommodate your baby's head at the birth, then a Caesarean delivery may well be indicated. It is worth noting, however, that the size of most babies is in proportion to the mothers who are carrying them.

Blood tests At your first appointment you will be asked to give a blood sample to confirm your blood group and to find out if you are Rh negative or positive. Your blood will also be checked to see if you are anemic and if you are immune to rubella (German measles). Other tests are also carried out to detect any serious conditions that could affect the development of your baby, such as syphilis and hepatitis B. If

WEEK 9: SPECIAL TESTS

Your blood will have been tested at your initial appointment to determine your blood group and to establish its Rh status. The Rh status of your blood depends on whether or not it possesses the Rh factor. If the factor is present, your blood is Rh-positive, if it is absent, your blood is Rh-negative. Most people's blood is Rh-positive.

If both you and the baby's father are Rh-negative, there is no problem. Complications only occur when the father's blood is Rh-positive and yours is Rh-negative. The unborn baby may acquire the Rh factor from its father, which can result in its blood being incompatible with yours. This can lead to a serious or even fatal illness for the baby before, or after the birth. Fortunately, this rarely affects a first pregnancy and it can be prevented in subsequent pregnancies by injections of Rhogan, an antibody that may be given during pregnancy and again within 72 hours of a baby being delivered.

SPECIAL TESTS

There are a number of prenatal tests that are used in special circumstances and usually only when there is some fear of genetic abnormality. They include:

Amniocentesis If you have a family history of genetic abnormalities such as Down's syndrome, cystic fibrosis, or spina bifida, or your blood shows a high or exceptionally low AFP (alpha-fetoprotein) level, you will be offered an amniocentesis, usually at around 16–18 weeks. This test is also offered to all women over 35 years of age because they have a

In an amniocentesis test the fetus's position is checked by ultrasound, before amniotic fluid is taken by a needle from the uterus.

higher risk of having a Down's syndrome baby. Guided by ultrasound scan, a long hollow needle is inserted through the wall of the abdomen and the uterus to draw out a sample of amniotic fluid. This is then tested for abnormalities. You will get the

You and your body

You will start putting on weight at this stage of your pregnancy. Your gums are becoming softer and thicker because of hormone changes so you will need to pay special attention to oral hygiene. Brush your teeth more frequently to avoid the risk of infections.

You should now familiarize yourself with some of the other prenatal procedures and tests that you can expect as your pregnancy progresses.

Your growing baby

The face is now developing well and the mouth and nose are now clearly visible. The limbs continue to grow rapidly and the fetus measures about 1¼ in.

results in about four weeks. The test carries a small risk of miscarriage.

Triple/double test This blood test is carried out at 16 weeks to measure the levels of three substances produced by the mother and the placenta. The levels change during pregnancy and a higher level could indicate that the baby may have Down's syndrome or spina bifida. The test cannot confirm that the baby is affected but it does indicate whether further tests, such as amniocentesis, are required. Not all doctors use the triple test; some offer the double test, where two substances are measured; others don't offer the test routinely, but you can ask to have it done.

Chorionic villus sampling (CVS) CVS is done at around 11 weeks to test for Down's syndrome or other genetic or chromosomal abnormalities. A fine tube is passed into the

Brush your teeth and gums regularly.

uterus to remove some of the cells from the tissue that surrounds the baby. The cells are then tested, and the results are usually known within one to two weeks. The advantage of CVS is that if the baby is found to have a problem and you want a termination it can be done early in pregnancy. However, there is a slightly higher risk of miscarriage with CVS than with amniocentesis.

Cordocentesis Very rarely done in the U.S., this test is administered to confirm diagnosis of chromosomal abnormalities and other handicaps, plus diseases such as rubella and toxoplasmosis. A hollow needle is inserted through the abdomen into the umbilical vein, close to the placenta, and a sample of the baby's blood is withdrawn. It is only performed after 18 weeks when the blood vessels are large enough. Results are usually known within about 48 hours.

GENETIC COUNSELING

If you are worried about the possibility of your children inheriting a disease or handicap, you can talk to a genetic counselor who is specially trained to help people with a family history of genetic disorders. Counseling is usually based on details of any genetic diseases that run in the family. A chromosome analysis from a blood sample may also be used. The counselor will be able to explain the likelihood of future children being affected by the genetic disorder and also about any tests that can be carried out. It is a good idea to have this discussion before attempting to get pregnant so that you know what is involved. Otherwise, tell your doctor that you want to see a genetic counselor when your pregnancy is confirmed.

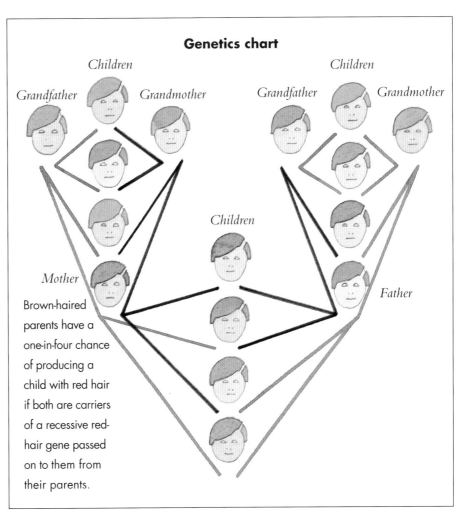

This genetics chart shows how red hair that is inherited through a recessive gene can miss a generation, but has a high chance of reappearing in the third generation. This can also apply to some inherited diseases.

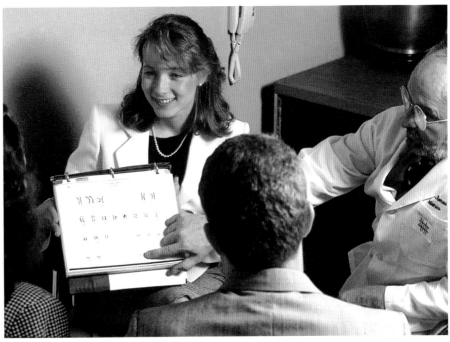

If your family has a history of a genetic disorder, you can talk to a genetic counselor who will discuss with you and your partner the likelihood of your baby having a problem.

WEEK 10: HORMONES/ HORMONAL CHANGES

Hormones play an important part during pregnancy and labor. The prime source of the hormones related to pregnancy are the ovaries during the early stages, and then the placenta once it is established at around 12 weeks. These hormones dictate how fast the fetus grows and are responsible for the changes in your breasts and body. They also ensure that your labor occurs at the right time.

High levels of the hormone called human chorionic gonadotrophin (HCG) circulate in your body during the first 12 weeks of pregnancy. They are responsible for any emotional changes, feeling tired, nausea, and vomiting.

HORMONES AND YOUR EMOTIONS
Pregnancy can produce a number of conflicting emotions, ranging from feelings of pure joy to bouts of black depression. It is quite natural to feel like this as you adjust to your changing role and come to terms with the fact that your life will never be quite the same again. You may find that you start worrying about whether you are ready for motherhood, or the effect that a new baby may have on your established relationship with your partner.

You may also find that mood swings, often brought on by the hormonal changes going on in your body, cause petty arguments between you. So it is most important

You and your body

There is an increase in the amount of blood that is circulating in your body, which may cause you to feel warmer than usual. Your uterus is now the size of a large orange and your changing shape may mean that you are more comfortable in loose-fitting clothes that do not restrict you.

Other changes are also taking place in your body. Although these are not always physically obvious, they are in fact the result of shifts in your body's chemistry.

Your growing baby

The external ears are now visible on the head, which is growing fast to make room for the brain. The fetal body is elongating and its fingers and toes are clearly defined but are still joined with webs of skin. At this stage of your pregnancy, the fetus is now about 1¾ in long and weighs around ¼ oz.

As you experience hormonal changes in your body you may find you become irritable and anxious. Discuss any of your worries with your partner who can talk things through with you and reassure you.

As your emotions are probably confused now, don't brood over heightened squabbles with your partner, but make up quickly.

If you find you're getting very tense, try practicing relaxation techniques on your own, or some deep breathing exercises.

Keep a personal record

Now that your pregnancy is confirmed and you have started planning your prenatal care and the type of birth you want to have, you may like to keep a record of your feelings and the physical changes that occur during your pregnancy. Useful things to include would be:

● Date of your last period, so that you can calculate your estimated delivery date (EDD) and then compare it with the actual birth date.

● Prenatal checks throughout your pregnancy.

● Prenatal tests and their results, along with the dates you were given them.

● The dates of scans which show your baby's development.

● Any foods that disagree with you, perhaps giving you indigestion.

● Ailments related to your pregnancy such as morning sickness and varicose veins.

● Your weight gain throughout the pregnancy.

● Your baby's first movement.

● Any drugs and medication including pain-relieving drugs during labor.

to make time to talk to each other so that you can both voice your feelings and share any worries or anxieties.

ASK YOUR DOCTOR TO EXPLAIN
It can often be difficult to remember everything that you are told at a check-up, so make notes of what your doctor tells you and don't be afraid to ask for an explanation of medical terms. Also write down any queries you may have beforehand, so that you don't forget to ask your doctor. The doctor will try to ensure that you understand the tests that you are being given.

WEEK 11: COMMON DISCOMFORTS

As your body prepares itself for birth, you may experience some physical effects. These are perfectly normal, can usually be dealt with easily, and should not leave any long-lasting effects, but knowing the reason for a complaint can often help in dealing with it.

Backache This can occur at any time, but usually happens when you try to compensate for your baby's weight by leaning backward which puts a strain on the lower back's muscles and joints. Try to avoid lifting heavy objects, bend with your knees bent, wear flat shoes, and always

Your back is now more vulnerable, so support it with a cushion when you sit down.

sit with your back well supported.

Bleeding gums Hormonal changes can cause a build-up of plaque on your teeth, which can

lead to bleeding gums. It is important to pay special attention to oral hygiene and to avoid snacking on sweets and sugary drinks. Dental treatment is especially important now so have at least two check-ups during this time.

Leg and foot cramps You may have a sudden sharp pain in your legs and feet, often at night. Try pulling your toes upward toward your ankles and rub the affected muscles. Regular gentle exercise will help prevent cramps.

Constipation Some of the extra hormones produced in pregnancy can cause the intestines to relax and become less efficient. Eating plenty of fruit, vegetables and fiber, and drinking water will help constipation.

You and your body

Any sickness should start to fade and you will begin to feel less tired than in the preceding weeks. You should start to think seriously about prenatal classes because they can get booked up quickly. Ask friends for referrals, or inquire at your doctor's office about local classes.

Fainting You may feel faint if you stand for too long or get up too quickly. This happens because not enough blood is getting to your brain; if the oxygen level gets too low you may actually faint. Try to rise slowly from either sitting or lying positions and, if you are standing, sit down and lower your head toward your knees.

Hemorrhoids These are a form of varicose vein that appear around the anus. They can be very uncomfortable as they are itchy and may even

Eating a high-fiber diet can help prevent painful constipation in pregnancy.

Your growing baby

Most of the major organs are formed, so the most vulnerable time will be over by the end of this week. The fetus is now relatively safe from any congenital abnormalities and infections, excepting rubella.

The external genitals have formed, along with either the ovaries or the testicles. The heart is now pumping blood to all the major organs of the body. The fetus weighs around ½ oz and is now about 2⅛ in long.

Although you may now be feeling less tired than in the early weeks, you should still rest as much as you can.

bleed slightly. If left untreated they can become prolapsed, which means they protrude through the anus, causing a good deal of pain. Eating high-fiber foods will keep your stools soft so that you don't have to strain, which puts pressure on hemorrhoids. An ice pack wrapped in a soft cloth, or a witch hazel compress, will bring relief, or you can buy a specially formulated hemorrhoid preparation from the pharmacist. Hemorrhoids usually disappear within a couple of weeks of the birth.

Vaginal discharge An increase in vaginal discharge during pregnancy is quite normal as long as the discharge is clear and white. If it becomes colored, smells, or makes you itchy, you may have developed an infection, such as yeast, which will need treatment.

Take some gentle, regular exercise with your partner as this will help to prevent leg cramps and keep you feeling fit.

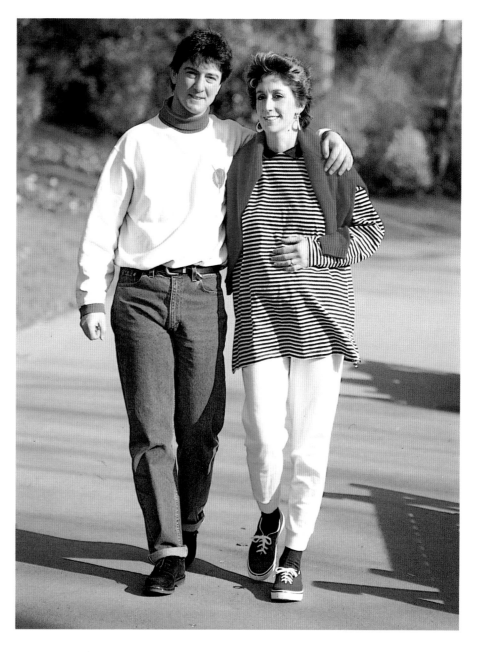

WEEK 12: HEALTHY EATING

The fetus gets all the nourishment it needs to grow from what you eat, so it is important to maintain a good diet throughout pregnancy. To achieve a healthy balanced diet you need to eat foods containing reasonable amounts of starchy carbohydrate, protein, fat, minerals, and vitamins each day. Starchy carbohydrates are found in bread, cereals, pasta, rice, and potatoes; they provide energy, vitamins, minerals, and fiber. Meat, fish, eggs, nuts, beans, peas, and lentils supply protein and minerals. Milk and dairy products such as hard cheese and yogurt will give you protein, vitamins, and calcium. Fresh fruit and vegetables and well-washed salads are good sources of minerals and vitamins. Folic acid can be found, along with other vitamins, in green leafy vegetables, fruit, nuts, bread, and rice.

If you are a vegetarian, you will need to increase your milk intake to at least 1 pint a day of either pasteurized milk or fortified soy milk, or the equivalent in cheese, yogurt, and dairy products.

Vegans will need to discuss their diet with a qualified dietitian as they could be deficient in calcium, iron, and vitamin B_{12}, which is found in foods of animal origin. Try to avoid

You and your body

You can expect to put on about one-quarter of your pregnancy weight between now and week 20. You may be beginning to feel more energetic and generally better than during the past few weeks. You should consider telling your employer at this time that you are pregnant.

Meanwhile, look at your lifestyle and be sure that your diet includes a sensible range of foods – for you and the unborn baby.

eating sugary snacks and carbonated drinks and keep "junk" foods to a minimum. Cut down on your caffeine intake from drinks like tea, coffee, chocolate and cola; try drinking bottled water and diluted fruit juices as alternatives.

Cut down on your caffeine levels and drink more diluted fruit juices.

Eat plenty of fruit when pregnant as it is a good source of minerals and vitamins.

A grain salad will give you plenty of fiber.

Vegetables are important in your pregnancy diet as they are low in fat and contain minerals, vitamins and folic acid in leafy varieties.

Use olive and light vegetable oils.

YOUR WEIGHT

Although you need extra energy during pregnancy to meet the needs of the developing fetus, and to store fat ready for breastfeeding later, you are not likely to need special energy foods. If you were an acceptable weight for your build before pregnancy, the only extra calories you should need are during the last three months when you eat around 200 extra calories a day. However, if you were overweight or underweight your weight gain will need monitoring, and a special diet may be necessary. Ask a professional for advice.

Your growing baby

The fetus's heart is beating at between 110 and 160 times a minute and its chest is beginning to rise and fall as it practices future breathing movements. Features are becoming more clearly defined and fingers and toes are now fully formed, with tiny nails beginning to grow. The fetus can suck its thumb and it swallows amniotic fluid and passes it back as urine. The amniotic fluid is completely replaced every 24 hours. The fetus is now about $2\frac{1}{2}$ in long and weighs $\frac{3}{4}$ oz.

WEEK 13: THE HEALTH PROFESSIONALS

You and your body
Your uterus is enlarging at a noticeable rate and you will be able to see the first signs of a visible belly. Your nipples have become darker and the blue veins in your breasts are a lot more obvious.

Now that you are at the end of the first trimester and your pregnancy is visible, you should start to familiarize yourself with some of the professionals with whom you will regularly be interacting.

During pregnancy, and after the birth, a number of different people will be involved in your care. How many you see will depend on where you are having your baby and the kind of prenatal care that is being offered. The type of professionals involved in your prenatal and post-partum care will be the same wherever you are having your baby.

Obstetrician-gynecologist (OB-GYN) In America, most women will receive their primary care, both before and during childbirth from an OB-GYN. Your doctor may be in private practice on his own, work with a partnership of other doctors, or be part of a health-maintenance organization (HMO). If there is more than one doctor involved in the practice, you should determine whether your care will be given by one primary physician or whether you will be treated by a number of different doctors, since this will certainly be a factor in your choice of practitioner.

It is more and more common in group practices for two or three OB-GYNs to take on patients in a rotation, so that each patient sees each doctor three or four times during the pregnancy. The doctors usually share similar opinions about procedures, medication, and treatments, but it is advisable to query each about your birth plan. The doctors divide up each 24-hour period so one is always on call, with the result that you will be assured of a familiar doctor when your time comes. Though perhaps it is preferable to see one doctor all the way through your pregnancy, if that doctor is off duty or away on vacation when you actually go into labor there is a chance that you might well end up with a complete stranger at your bedside.

Certified nurse-midwife An increasing choice among women looking for less medicalized, more personal births, a nurse-midwife has been trained to be an expert in pregnancy and labor. She can offer prenatal care, or you can see a physician for prenatal care and utilize the midwife during labor and delivery. When considering a midwife, make sure to ask if she is associated with a physician; this can be very important if any risks develop during pregnancy or childbirth.

Some midwives work in a kind of group practice called a maternity center, which is generally associated with one or more physicians who are called on for consultations when it is necessary. Maternity centers offer not only full prenatal care but facilities for labor and delivery. Be aware, however, that you may have to be transferred from the maternity-center to a hospital should your birth

As your pregnancy progresses you may be examined by an obstetrician who specializes in birth and child care. She will advise on your baby's development and discuss any problems.

Your growing baby

The fetus is now 3 in long and weighs 1½ oz. The bone marrow, liver, and spleen have now taken over production of blood cells. The bones are developing and the teeth are in place. The fetus may already be practicing lip movements to develop the muscles needed for the sucking reflex after the birth.

The pediatrician will perform several checks on your baby after birth. Here he is checking that the newborn's foot reflex works correctly.

be considered or become high-risk.

Most hospitals have a group of midwives who are available to attend labor and delivery in the hospital rooms. If you want to use a midwife this can be the best of both worlds as you will have the hospital's technology to call on if any complications suddenly arise.

High-risk practitioner Also known as neonatalogists or maternal-fetal specialists, these physicians work with women whose pregnancies have been labeled "high-risk." They may consult with a woman's regular OB-GYN or actually take over as the primary physician. If you have reason to believe that your pregnancy is in the high-risk category, you may well want to consider consulting a specialist in the early weeks at the beginning of your pregnancy.

Pediatrician This is a doctor who specializes in caring for babies and children. Your baby will have a complete check-up by a pediatrician soon after the birth.

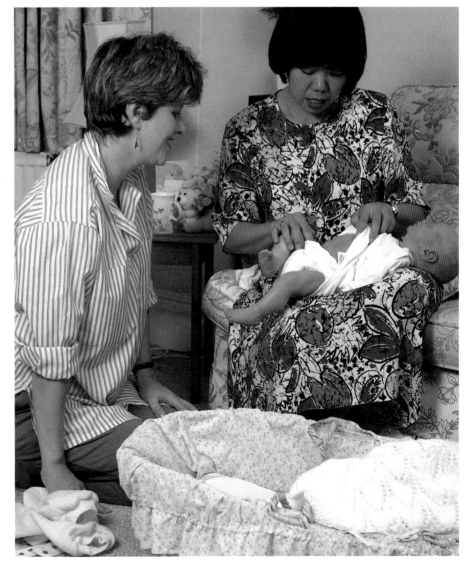

After your baby's birth his navel will need to be checked to ensure that it is healing.

THE SECOND TRIMESTER

WEEK 14: SEX DURING PREGNANCY

To be able to enjoy sex it is important to know that making love cannot harm the developing fetus. It is well protected in the uterus by the amniotic fluid and membranes, and the uterus itself is sealed with a plug of mucus, which stays in place until just before the birth. Even deep penetration is safe, but it should of course be gentle so that it doesn't cause discomfort.

Many women find that the middle months of pregnancy are a sensual and even erotic time. Physical changes, such as the increase in the size of your breasts, can actually serve to heighten your interest in sex, which in turn leads to an increase in sexual pleasure. Your genitals may also appear bigger and the pressure from the growing baby can actually make them more responsive. Some women find that they experience orgasm for the first time during pregnancy, while others come to orgasm much more quickly.

Experiencing orgasm is perfectly safe; in fact it can be considered to be beneficial since the uterus often remains hard and firm for several minutes afterward. This is similar in effect to the Braxton Hicks, or practice, contractions you experience toward the end of your pregnancy that prepare the uterus for the birth of your baby.

You may of course find that you feel a lessening of desire during pregnancy, or even a complete loss of interest in sex. These feelings are not uncommon, but they can cause unnecessary stress between you and your partner if they are not brought out into the open and discussed.

You and your body

You are now beginning the second trimester when you should start experiencing what is known as mid-pregnancy bloom. You will be feeling better about everything; if your sex drive has diminished over the last few months it will probably return and sex may be better than ever.

If you don't feel much like making love in early pregnancy, still cuddle your partner and show him lots of affection.

Your partner may feel that he is being rejected, so it is important to find alternative ways of giving each other love and reassurance.

DIFFERENT WAYS TO MAKE LOVE
It is important that you and your partner show each other physical affection during pregnancy, but this does not always have to involve sexual intercourse. You may find as your pregnancy progresses that you want lots of cuddles and other signs of affection from your partner without actually having sex. Men often find this hard to understand as they tend to link such physical contact with intercourse. Explain to your partner how you feel so that together you can find other ways of expressing your love for each other.

Try experimenting with different forms of sex play that don't necessarily end in penetration, so that you can still make love even if you don't feel like intercourse. Take time to

Often during the middle months of pregnancy, you can start to feel more sensual and show renewed interest in sex.

find out what you both enjoy and don't be afraid to tell your partner what you do and don't like.

Stroking, massage, mutual masturbation, and oral sex are some alternative ways of making love that you can both enjoy and that may at times be more appropriate than full intercourse.

As you grow larger you'll find some positions for lovemaking more comfortable than others. Experiment with positions that keep your partner's weight off you.

USING SEX TO INDUCE LABOR
Sex can sometimes be a way of

inducing labor. Your partner's semen contains a hormone called prostaglandin, which will help to soften the cervix in preparation for birth. Lovemaking will also stimulate the cells in the cervix to secrete their own prostaglandins; this too may help bring labor on.

Breast stimulation in late pregnancy sometimes produces quite strong contractions which are thought to help prepare the way for labor by softening and drawing up the cervix. It has been discovered that stimulating nipples can reactivate a labor that has halted – something that your partner might like to remember.

Your growing baby

The fetus is beginning to look human as the chin, forehead, and nose become more clearly defined. It can now turn its head around and even wrinkle its brow. The fetus may even respond to external stimulus by actually moving away when the doctor or midwife examines your abdomen. The fetus is now 3½ in long and weighs about 2 oz.

WEEK 15: HEALTH AND SAFETY

You may hear about risks during pregnancy. Some are valid, others are based on misinformation.

If you work with dangerous substances such as chemicals or in a job that requires you to do heavy lifting, you could be risking your health and the health of your child. Your employer must offer you an alternative job if yours is a recognized risk. If you are concerned about risks at work talk to your doctor, your employer, or union representative.

A common concern among working women is that sitting all day in front of a VDT screen such as a computer terminal or word processor will harm the developing fetus. The most recent research shows no evidence of this being a risk, but you may need to have your microwave checked out for any minor radiation leaks, although with modern equipment these are very unlikely.

You and your body

Your heart has enlarged to cope with the increased amount of blood circulating in your body and the fetus's need for oxygen, and has increased its output by 20 percent. You will be feeling more energetic than before and now is a good time to take a vacation before the birth.

HEALTH HAZARDS

While you are pregnant you should avoid unpasteurized milk and products made with unpasteurized milk; pâté made from meat, fish, or vegetables; soft and blue vein cheeses; pre-cooked poultry; and prepared salads (unless they are washed thoroughly) because of the risk of listeria.

Listeria monocytogenes is the bacterium which causes listeriosis in humans and animals. Animals that carry the bacterium are likely to infect the milk they produce and the meat that is produced from them. The bacterium is usually destroyed during the pasteurization of milk and milk products. However, if food is contaminated and then refrigerated the bacteria will continue to multiply. Listeriosis can also be spread through direct contact with animals that are infected.

Toxoplasmosis is a disease that occurs in both humans and animals. It can be extremely dangerous if it is contracted during pregnancy because it may cause miscarriage or severe fetal abnormality. The disease is spread to humans by eating undercooked or raw meat and through coming into contact with cat feces. As it is quite possible to have the disease without knowing it, you should have a blood test to find out whether

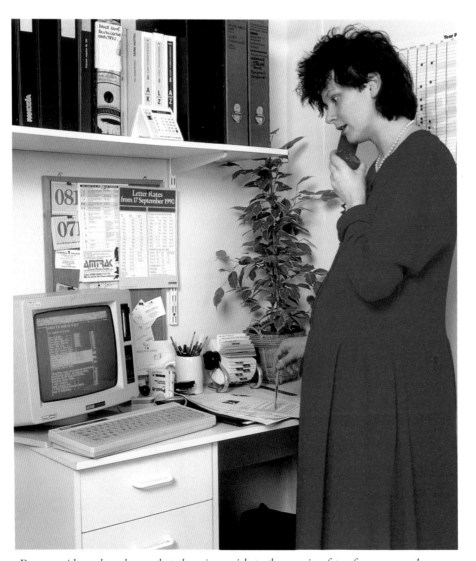

Recent evidence has shown that there is no risk to the growing fetus for women who regularly use computer terminals. However, move around often to minimize backache.

The fetal skeleton is developing well and its legs are now longer than its arms. The hair on its head is becoming thicker and it has eyelashes as well as eyebrows. The fetus can probably hear now and the amniotic fluid makes an excellent sound conductor, so it will be able to hear your stomach rumbling and your heart beating as well as the sound of your voice. The fetus is 4¾ in long and now weighs 3½ oz.

or not you have immunity. If you are immune, you definitely cannot infect your baby.

If you find that you are not immune, you should take a number of precautions throughout your pregnancy. Avoid any meat that has not been cooked thoroughly and wash your hands, cooking utensils, and surfaces after preparing raw meat. Wash fruit and vegetables to remove all traces of dirt. Avoid unpasteurized goats' milk and goats' milk products. Finally, always wear rubber gloves when gardening and wash your hands well afterward. Put covers on your children's sand boxes in the yard to prevent any cats from getting in them and using them as litter boxes. Finally, always wear some rubber gloves when handling used cat litter, and remember to wash your hands and also the gloves when you have finished.

Above: Hard cheeses are safe to eat in pregnancy. However, make sure you only eat hard-boiled eggs and drink pasteurized milk to avoid Listeria monocytogenes. *Right: Always wear some gloves when gardening during pregnancy as toxoplasmosis can be caught from cat feces.*

Food safety

Avoid putting yourself at risk during pregnancy by taking the following precautions with food.
● Wash all fruit, vegetables, and salads, including any pre-packaged salads, thoroughly.
● Don't eat raw or undercooked meat.
● Eggs must be well cooked and all dairy products should be pasteurized.
● Avoid eating any soft, imported cheeses such as Brie and Camembert, blue-vein cheeses, and those that are made from goats' and sheep's milk because of the risk of listeria.
● Don't eat liver and liver products, such as pâté and liverwurst. They contain high levels of vitamin A, which is toxic in excessive amounts.
● Avoid shellfish.
● Keep your refrigerator below 41°F and don't refreeze any previously frozen foods.
● Pay special attention to hygiene in the kitchen.
● Don't eat food that is past its expiration date.

WEEK 16: SCANS/TWINS

At around 16 weeks you may be offered an ultrasound scan so that you can see your baby for the first time. A scan can be carried out at any stage of pregnancy, but is usually offered between 16 and 20 weeks.

The procedure is completely painless. High-density sound waves are used to create a picture of your baby in the uterus, and you will be able to see this on a screen. The best pictures are obtained when you have a full bladder so you will be asked to drink a lot of fluid beforehand.

You lie on a table and your stomach is lubricated so that the person performing the scan can pass the scanner smoothly across it. The picture that appears on the screen may not be very clear, so ask the sonographer to explain the rather indistinct images to you, if you are unsure of anything that you are seeing.

The fetus's age can be determined from a scan; it also shows up most abnormalities of the head and spine that may have occurred and will detect the presence of twins. The exact position of the placenta and the fetus can be seen, so if there are any problems, for example when the placenta is situated very low down, extra care will be taken throughout your pregnancy.

TWINS

There is about a one in 80 chance that you and your partner will conceive twins. However, you are more likely to give birth to twins if you have a history of them in your, or your partner's, family.

Identical twins come from one egg which, once fertilized, then splits into two separate cells. Each of the cells then grows into a separate fetus, but they usually share the same placenta. Because identical twins originally came from the same cells they are always the same sex and look like each other.

Non-identical twins, also known as fraternal twins, are the result of two eggs being fertilized by two

You and your body

You may feel your baby's first movements around this time. These early movements are like a fluttering, bubbling sensation. You may notice the beginning of *Linea nigra*, a dark line that appears down the center of your abdomen. This will disappear after the birth.

different sperm at the same time. Each fetus has its own placenta and the sexes of the babies may differ.

Fraternal twins usually don't look any more alike than brothers and sisters who are born years apart.

An ultrasound scan may be carried out around your 16th week of pregnancy. It will show up abnormalities in your baby and also indicate the presence of twins.

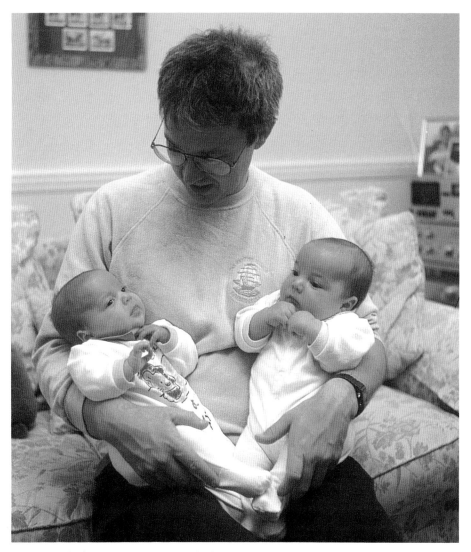

The arrival of twins can come as a shock. Get your partner to help as much as he can and you will soon find that you both start bonding with them.

Your growing baby

The fetus will be moving around frequently now, although you may have only just started to feel these movements. The body will become covered in a fine downy hair called lanugo. It is possible to tell a baby's sex now through an ultrasound scan, though scans aren't 100-percent effective as predictors of gender. The fetus is 6¼ in long and weighs 5 oz.

Twins in the womb

Fraternal twins

Identical twins

The joy of having twins is that as they grow up they will learn to play with each other.

WEEK 17: YOUR PREGNANCY WARDROBE

You will find that loose ordinary clothes, in a bigger size if necessary, will see you through most of your pregnancy. A few basic garments that are interchangeable will help you achieve a variety of looks. Buy skirts and slacks with elasticated waists, baggy shirts, and big T-shirts in natural fibers such as cotton. Choose underwear with some cotton content for softness and absorbency and maternity tights or stockings to give your legs support. As your breasts are likely to increase in size rapidly during the early months of pregnancy, it makes sense to buy a well-fitting support bra early. This will prevent your breasts from sagging which will help them to return to their normal shape once the baby is born.

You and your body

Your waistline will have completely disappeared and you may have begun to develop stretch marks. Bleeding gums may be a problem, so if you haven't had a dental check-up now is the time to go. If you work, you should start thinking about when you intend to leave and whether you will want to return.

Your growing baby

All your baby's limbs are now fully formed as well as the skin and muscle. Its taste buds are beginning to develop so that it will be able to distinguish sweet from non-sweetened fluid. The fetus is now about 7 in long and weighs around 6½ oz.

Maternity benefits

Once your pregnancy is confirmed, you should make inquiries about your maternity benefits. If you work you may qualify for maternity leave from your employer. You may be allowed to take time off work to attend prenatal classes. Your obstetrician or midwife will help or advise if you are unsure of what to do. Check your health-insurance policy to determine what benefits are and aren't covered. Under the new Family Leave act all companies with over 50 employees must grant 12 weeks of unpaid leave, except to those in the top 10% income bracket (they assume you are too essential to take up that much time so it's discretionary). Negotiate leave and compensation early to avoid any confusion.

A baggy cardigan worn over a skirt with an elasticated waist helps conceal your belly.

A loose-fitting pants suit with a long jacket can look and feel good in pregnancy.

Front-opening dresses won't be restricting, and can be useful for breastfeeding.

If your feet ache take off your shoes inside your home, but be careful on polished surfaces.

You can still stay fashionable by wearing a larger size of leggings over your belly, which can be concealed with a long, loose T-shirt.

Front-opening clothes are comfortable to wear in both early and late pregnancy, as they expand with you.

WEEK 18: LOOKING YOUR BEST

You may find that your hair behaves in a rather unpredictable way while you are pregnant. Hormone changes mean that your hair may appear thicker than usual, or in some women the opposite happens and the hair loss increases so that the hair looks thinner. Dry hair may become even drier and oily hair more greasy. Whichever condition applies to you, just wash your hair using a mild shampoo. If your hair tends to be very dry, use a good conditioner after every wash and, if possible, allow it to dry naturally rather than using a hair dryer.

Dry hair will need extra conditioning during your pregnancy because it becomes drier as your hormones change.

Pregnancy hormones can affect the color and texture of your skin. Uneven patches appear and dark-skinned people may even get a but-

Try using hypoallergenic skin-cleansing products on your skin as it will be particularly sensitive at this time.

terfly-shaped patch of pigmentation across the face known as "the mask of pregnancy." A heavier foundation will help hide these marks and a UVA sun screen will prevent any further increase in pigmentation. Pregnancy "bloom," which is caused by an increase in the tiny blood vessels under the surface of the skin, can be toned down with green cream or powder. It is a good idea to use hypoallergenic skin-care products as your skin may be particularly sensitive at this time.

FLUID RETENTION

Your body retains more water than usual during pregnancy, so your hands and feet may become slightly swollen and you may find that your eyes get puffy and your face looks

You and your body

You should be able to feel the fetal movements quite clearly now. Your nose may become blocked as pregnancy causes the membranes inside the nasal passages to swell. You may also notice an increase in vaginal discharge. You will find that there are several physical changes besides the predictable weight gain.

fuller. The best solution is to get as much rest as possible, sitting with your feet higher than your heart, as this will help reduce the swelling in your feet and ankles. While you are resting, place some cotton pads soaked in witch hazel, or slices of cucumber, on your eyes. This will soothe them and reduce any puffiness. You can disguise a fuller face by applying blusher below the cheekbones and blending a darker shade of foundation along your jawline. Alternatively, you can draw attention away from your face by wearing a colorful scarf or a chunky necklace around your neck.

Try not to be too critical of your changing looks during pregnancy; many other people will consider that this new, softer look to your appearance makes you seem altogether younger and healthier.

Your growing baby

The skin is still wrinkled because the fetus hasn't started to gain body fat and is very active. It is becoming aware of sounds outside the uterus and you may be able to feel it jumping at unexpected noises. The fetus is now around 8½ in long and weighs about 8 oz.

With extra care you can transform your face from looking tired and pale in pregnancy (left) to attractive and striking (right). A concealing foundation masks any pigmentation marks, mascara and soft eye shadows can highlight your eyes, and a vivid lipstick can emphasize your mouth.

WEEK 19: EXERCISE

Regular, gentle exercise has an important part to play in keeping you fit during pregnancy and will help you get back into shape after the birth. Remember, if you ever feel faint, light-headed or breathless while you are exercising you must stop immediately. If you haven't been exercising regularly, start swimming, or take up yoga or walking as

they can all be done at a gentle, rhythmic pace that can be adapted to suit each stage of your pregnancy. If you find it easier to follow an exercise routine you can do at home, never include sit-ups or exercises that involve raising the legs when you are lying down as these could damage the abdominal muscles. It is important to stop and relax between

You and your body

You have started to put weight on your buttocks, hips, and thighs as well as your abdomen. Tiny veins may start appearing on your face. These are very small broken blood vessels which are caused by circulation changes. They will disappear after the birth.

exercises and to make sure that your breathing always remains at a controlled rate.

Toning your breasts

1 *Hold arms at breast level with hands loosely clasping opposite arm. Tighten grip and hold briefly, then relax.*

2 *Still keeping your hands clasped, raise them to eye level and tighten your grip and hold, then relax.*

3 *Lower your arms to your waist, tighten and hold, then relax. Repeat this sequence several times.*

Feet exercises

1 *To loosen ankles, sit down with feet flat on the ground. Lift one foot at a time and circle ankle five times in both directions.*

2 *To tone the feet, place your feet flat on the floor. Now lift your toes up as far as you can and hold briefly, then relax.*

3 *Now clench your toes hard, hold for a few seconds, then relax again. Repeat this technique, and Step 2, 10 times.*

Taylor sitting and squatting exercises

1 *To loosen the groin and hips and stretch the inner thighs, sit with the soles of your feet together. Holding ankles, bring your pelvis and feet together by moving your hips toward your feet.*

2 *This is a good position for labor. Squat down keeping a straight back; try to put your heels down placing your weight evenly. Press your elbows against your thighs stretching the inner groin and thighs.*

Tummy toning exercises

1 *Put a folded towel or pillow under your head and lie with your knees bent and your feet flat on the floor. Press the small of your back down on the floor.*

2 *Slowly extend both your legs in front of you until they are both completely straight, but still keep your back pressed well down onto the floor.*

Your growing baby

The fetus is starting to put on weight and its rapid rate of growth has begun to slow down. The baby teeth have developed in the gums and the buds for the permanent teeth are beginning to form. The fetus is around 9 in long and weighs about 10 oz.

3 *Draw one knee up and then the other, without lifting your back off the floor. Relax your legs until straight; repeat five times.*

WEEK 20: SKIN CARE/CRAVINGS

Your breasts are likely to increase by as much as two bra sizes during pregnancy, so you will need to make sure that they are well supported so that they do not sag and become uncomfortable. Small bumps may appear in the skin around your nipples. These are sebaceous glands that secrete sebum, a fatty lubricant. As your pregnancy progresses, your nipples grow softer and gentle massage will help make them supple and ready for breastfeeding. Your breasts may leak a yellow fluid called colostrum, which will form a crust on the nipples. You will need to wash and dry them gently and thoroughly at least twice a day.

Your nails are made of protein and are affected by the hormonal changes taking place in your body. Usually they grow longer and stronger during pregnancy, but occasionally pregnancy will cause them to split and break. If this happens, keep them short and protect them by wearing gloves when you are doing rough jobs or when you immerse your hands in water.

If the elasticity of your skin becomes overstretched as you put on

Your nails may be brittle during pregnancy so keep them short to stop them splitting.

Check your bra size by measuring around your ribcage. For cup size measure around your bust at its fullest.

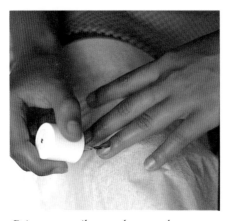

Paint on a nail strengthener to keep your nails strong at this time.

You and your body

Your uterus is enlarging quite rapidly now so that you look pregnant. Your navel may be flattened or pushed out and it will stay this way until after the birth. Heartburn may start to become a problem because the uterus is starting to push against your stomach.

weight, you may develop stretch marks. These usually appear on the breasts, stomach, and the tops of the thighs as thin, reddish lines. There is little you can do to avoid them, but keeping your skin well moisturized, and being careful not to put on too much extra weight, will help minimize them. Stretch marks fade to thin silvery lines after the birth.

Varicose veins can be caused by pregnancy hormones or, later in pregnancy, by the uterus pressing down and obstructing the flow of blood from the legs to the heart. Although not serious, they can lead to aching or sore legs. Try to avoid standing for long periods and put your feet up whenever possible to ease any discomfort. Walking will help the blood flow; put on support tights or stockings when you get out of bed in the morning to give your legs more support. Varicose veins usually disappear soon after the birth.

CRAVINGS

No one is sure why some pregnant women have cravings while others don't. Doctors disagree about them; some are sympathetic while others doubt that they actually exist. If you desire a certain food there is no reason why you shouldn't indulge yourself within reason, but make sure that you don't exclude other more nourishing foods as a result.

Above: Your legs may ache more with the increased weight you're carrying, so try massaging them with a pleasant body lotion. Right: You can't prevent stretch marks from appearing on your stomach, but rubbing in lotion may help to reduce them.

Your growing baby

Vernix, a white greasy substance, is starting to form over the fetus's skin to protect it from the amniotic fluid. This usually wears off before the birth, but sometimes traces of it can be seen. At this stage in your pregnancy the fetus weighs around 12 oz and measures about 10 in.

WEEK 21: MINOR COMPLAINTS

You and your body

You should be able to see your abdomen ripple as the fetus moves. You may be feeling slightly breathless as your expanding ribcage pushes upward, giving your lungs less room. You will probably be feeling energetic so now is the time to tackle things such as planning the baby's room.

By now you may be experiencing some of the minor problems that occur later in pregnancy. These include:

Heartburn This is a strong burning feeling in your chest that often happens during the last few months of pregnancy. It is usually worse when lying down. Hormones cause the valve at the top of your stomach to relax, which allows stomach acid to pass back into the esophagus, causing a burning sensation. Avoid eating spicy and fatty foods. Eating small, but frequent meals may help reduce heartburn. Sleeping propped up at night and drinking a glass of milk before you go to bed may also help ease the discomfort. Your

pharmacist that you are pregnant because some of the remedies available are not suitable for use during pregnancy or breastfeeding.

Insomnia Sleeplessness often

If you are suffering from heartburn, try drinking a glass of milk before you go to sleep at night.

doctor may prescribe an antacid if the problem regularly keeps you awake at night. If you buy an over-the-counter remedy always tell the

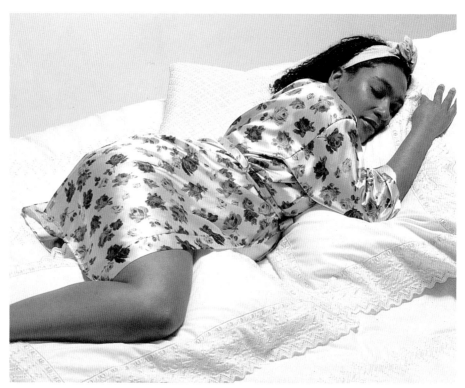

Insomnia can be a problem in later pregnancy. If you can't sleep, try supporting your tummy on pillows to make yourself more comfortable.

becomes a problem as your pregnancy progresses because you find it difficult to get comfortable, and you have to make frequent trips to the bathroom. Vivid dreams can also be a problem at this time. A bath followed by a warm drink at bedtime will help you relax. It is important to find restful sleeping positions, so use lots of pillows to support your abdomen when you lie on your side. You could also try practicing some relaxation techniques.

Itching This often occurs on the

areas of skin around the belly and is sometimes accompanied by a rash. Calamine lotion should help relieve the itching and since it is usually caused by sweating, wearing loose clothes made of natural fibers can help prevent it. Severe itching during the last three months of pregnancy could be a warning of pregnancy cholestasis – a rare but potentially dangerous liver disorder – and you should consult your doctor.

Edema (swelling) This occurs in the feet and ankles and sometimes

Your growing baby

The fetus is very active now and you will probably be able to feel it kicking quite easily. If this disturbs you at night, stroke your tummy and talk to the fetus because it may be soothed by the sound of your voice. The fetus is now around 11 in long and weighs about 14 oz.

the hands because your body is retaining more fluid than normal. By the end of the day this fluid tends to gather in your feet, especially if the weather has been hot or you have been doing a lot of standing. Try to sit or lie with your feet up whenever you can, as this will help reduce the swelling. Wear support hose and comfortable shoes during the day and avoid standing for long periods. You should always tell your doctor about any swelling that you experience as it may possibly be a sign of preeclampsia.

Fatigue The extra weight you carry during late pregnancy can make you feel more tired than usual. It is important to build some regular rest periods into your day when you

can sit down with your feet up. If the fatigue you are experiencing feels excessive, you may be suffering from anemia. Make sure you are getting plenty of iron in your diet by eating lean red meat, whole grains, dark green leafy vegetables, nuts, and legumes. If the feeling still persists then ensure you consult your doctor.

Above: You may well be feeling more energetic than usual at this stage in your pregnancy, but don't forget to give yourself time to sit down and rest.

Below: If your ankles start to swell when you have been on your feet for a while, lie down on the floor with your head supported by a pillow and your feet propped up on several pillows.

WEEK 22: RELAXATION AND MASSAGE

It is important to be able to relax, both mentally and physically, during pregnancy because this will help you to rest. Knowing how to make your body relax during labor will allow you to work with the contractions rather than against them.

Physical relaxation
Start by getting comfortable and make sure that every part of your body is supported. Then concentrate on tensing and relaxing individual parts of your body. Start at your toes and work gradually upward to your head and then back down to your toes again. By the time you have finished this exercise you should be feeling nice and loose.

Mental relaxation This requires deep concentration so you need to be completely comfortable and in a quiet place where no one will disturb you. Empty your mind and concentrate on your breathing. Breathe in deeply and hold your breath for a few seconds before letting it out slowly. Once you have established a steady

You and your body
Your lower ribs are starting to cause you pain as they get pushed outward by your growing baby and your expanding uterus. Your ribcage rises by a small amount as it is pushed upward. To minimize the discomfort, try sitting up as straight as you can or lifting your arms above your head. This is an ideal time to investigate the different methods that you can use to ease discomfort now and during labor and birth.

pattern of breathing you should make sure that all your muscles are relaxed, then allow your mind to float away. One way to do this is to imagine that you are floating gently on calm water under a clear blue sky, in tranquil surroundings.

OTHER TECHNIQUES

Massage is an excellent way of relieving tension. It is best done on bare skin, but if you find your skin is particularly sensitive, it can be carried out through a thin cotton nightgown. Massage strokes should be firm, smooth, and rhythmic.

Aromatherapy massage uses essential oils that are added to a carrier oil before being applied to your skin. Certain essential oils can be dangerous during pregnancy because they may trigger uterine contractions, so you must always get qualified professional advice. Many aromatherapists will not treat a pregnant woman at all. Most of those who will treat expectant mothers will do so only after the sixth month of pregnancy. One effective blend is mandarin oil well diluted (i.e. a maximum solution of one percent: no more than 10 drops of oil to 50 ml carrier oil) in a sweet almond carrier oil. A well-diluted solution of true lavender, jasmine, and rose in sweet almond oil is also thought to be beneficial during labor and birth.

In acupuncture tiny needles are

used to stimulate meridian points situated on the body's energy lines with the aim of rebalancing the energy flow. The treatment can help backache, but some points on the body are thought to stimulate uterine contractions, so it is important to visit a qualified practitioner and let him or her know that you are pregnant.

Above: If you are suffering regularly from backache, having a soothing massage from a qualified practitioner can help. With an aromatherapy massage, make sure she chooses oils that will not affect the baby.

Below: Regular massage on your legs may help to relieve any aches and pains that you are experiencing.

WEEK 23: PREPARING THE BABY'S ROOM

This is a good time to think of practical things like planning the baby's room. Whether you have a spare room which you are going to turn into a baby's room, or you intend to make a corner for your baby in your own bedroom, you should start getting it ready now while you still have the energy.

Before you begin you will need to take into consideration the shape and size of the area so you can decide how much furniture and baby equipment will comfortably fit into it. You should also check whether there are enough electrical sockets; that there is sufficient heating and that the ceiling or wall lights are

where you want them. Major changes such as rewiring or putting in another radiator are better done before you start to decorate or carpet the baby's room.

Babies enjoy looking at bright, primary colors and big, bold patterns so choose a colorful paint and paper; washable materials will make it easier to keep the walls looking bright and fresh. Decals, borders, pictures, and mobiles can be used very effectively to brighten up a plain background if you are reluctant to commit yourself to a color scheme until you know your baby's sex.

Rugs and polished floors look nice but are unsuitable because of

You and your body

The baby can now be felt through your abdominal wall and the doctor will palpate your abdomen to see how the baby is lying. You may occasionally feel a pain that is rather like a stitch down the side of your stomach. This is the uterine muscle stretching and it will go away after you have had a rest.

the risk of slipping on them while holding the baby. Any flooring needs to be warm underfoot and non-slip. Sealed cork tiles are ideal because they are warm and any spills can be wiped up without damage to the floor. Fitted carpets and carpet tiles are suitable alternatives, but don't buy expensive carpet because it will probably need replacing after a relatively short time.

An overhead light with a dimmer switch or a specially designed baby's room light is very useful for night feeding as it gives out a soft comforting glow that won't startle either of you too much in the middle of the night. A nightlight will provide enough illumination for you to check on your sleeping baby, but you will need a brighter light for diaper changing and general care. Avoid any lamps with trailing cords that you could trip over, and fit all unused electrical sockets with a safety cover.

FINISHING TOUCHES

The room where the baby sleeps must be draft-proof so cover any windows with thick, lined curtains. These will not only keep out the cold but will also keep the morning light from waking your baby during the summer. Windows need to be

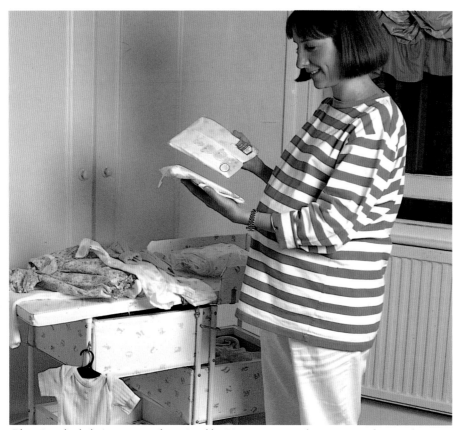

Planning the baby's room can be enjoyable. You can start to buy some outfits in advance, but remember that you will often be given baby clothes when your baby is born.

fitted with childproof locks and the curtains should be out of reach of the crib. Never place the baby's crib under a window or near radiators. Young babies cannot regulate their own temperature so they need to be kept in a comfortably warm environment at around a constant 65°F. A special baby's room thermometer or a thermostat fitted to the radiator will help ensure that you maintain the room temperature.

Babies actually require very little in the way of furniture. Somewhere to sleep, a dresser or chest to keep clothes in, and a place for changing and storing toiletries and diapers, as well as a chair for you to sit in while you are feeding or rocking the baby, is all that you really need for the first few months. All baby's room furniture should be sturdy enough that it can't be pulled over when babies are older and using it for support as they

begin to pull themselves up onto their feet.

If you buy secondhand furniture, make sure that any paint or varnish is non-toxic and lead-free. Also check that there are no broken bits to harm your baby. Unless you're sure that the crib conforms to current safety standards, don't buy it.

Your growing baby

The fetus is beginning to look as it will at birth, with the head much more in proportion to the body. In a boy, the scrotum is now well developed and in a girl the ovaries already contain several million eggs. (These will reduce to around two million at birth and will continue decreasing until puberty is reached.) The fetus is around 12¼ in long and weighs approximately 15½ oz.

When decorating your baby's room, bear in mind that babies like bright, primary colors. They also love pretty mobiles.

A basket can by kept by or near your bed, and your baby can sleep in it for up to three months.

WEEK 24: BABY CLOTHES AND EQUIPMENT

Start planning what you need to buy for your baby so that by the birth you will at least have purchased the major items. If you leave everything until the end of the pregnancy, you may be too tired to enjoy shopping for your baby.

Only buy a few basic first size or newborn garments as your baby will probably rapidly outgrow these. Also, most baby clothes are sized by the approximate age and height of the child and you won't know the size of your child until she is born.

Choose some well-designed baby clothes, which will make your life easier and allow you to dress and undress your baby with the minimum of time and fuss. Clothes with elastic necks or a shoulder fastening will let you slip clothes over the

baby's head easily, and snaps up the inside of legs of rompers or stretchies will help to ease the regular diaper changing that is necessary.

Your new baby will probably go through as many as three changes of clothes a day, so it is a good idea to check the washing instructions on any garment before you buy. These instructions will tell you how best to care for each garment so that you

You and your body

You will noticeably be putting on weight, perhaps as much as 1 lb per week. Your feet and legs may start to feel the strain of carrying this extra weight, so make sure that you wear comfortable shoes and that you get plenty of rest.

can see whether it is easy-care, or if it will require a lot of attention.

BABY'S TRANSPORT
Before you decide on a carriage, stroller or combination, you need to consider your lifestyle and the various methods of transport you will be

A baby's layette: a hat, undershirt, stretchie, mittens, booties, diaper and a cardigan.

Baby transport

Transportation choices include a carriage (left) or a folding stroller (right).

A traditional carriage is sturdy with plenty of space to carry shopping. It is probably the best option if you walk everywhere and you are planning to have another child fairly quickly. Generally, carriages are unsuitable for cars unless they are fitted with a detachable body.

A folding stroller with a reclining seat can be used from babyhood through to toddler stage. Choose one that is light enough to carry on and off public transportation.

A stroller that converts to a carriage is especially useful, as is a lightweight umbrella stroller.

A folding stroller with a package shelf can be very useful when you go shopping with your baby.

using regularly. You also need to think about where it will be stored when not in use. Once you have selected the type most suitable to your needs, see if the store you order it from will keep it for you until after the baby is born.

When buying a car seat, you can choose between an infant carrier, which is suitable from birth to six months, or a combination seat, which is suitable from birth to around four years. Both types are held securely in place using the existing car seat belts.

EQUIPMENT

Whether you buy a crib, basket, or bassinette will probably depend on where your baby is going to sleep and how much space you have available. If the baby is going to sleep in your room at first and you haven't much space, think about buying a crib later.

However, when you do purchase a crib make sure that the new mat-

Your growing baby

Vigorous movements followed by periods of quiet will start to occur as the fetus develops its own waking and resting periods. The pattern that develops now may well continue after the birth so it's a good idea to monitor it for a few days to see how it compares with the sleep pattern once the baby is born. The heartbeat can be heard with an ordinary stethoscope and the fetus can hear you clearly when you speak. It is now around 13 in long and weighs about 1 lb.

tress you get to go in it is firm. It should also fit snugly into the base of the crib.

You need to have at least six sheets and several lightweight blankets for the crib and another six sheets and at least three more blankets for your carriage or stroller. You may want to include a crib bumper and comforter as well.

A car seat carrier is easily transported and can be bought in different sizes to suit the age of your baby.

A two-level high chair can be used in the higher position when your baby is young (left) and in the lower position (above) when he is older. Always make sure you strap him in securely.

WEEK 25: FEEDING CHOICES

You should be looking rosy-cheeked and healthy because of the increase in blood circulation under the skin. Pressure from the growing uterus on the bladder means that you need to make frequent trips to the bathroom. Leg cramps, heartburn, and backache are often problems now.

Now is the time to start thinking about how you are going to feed your baby. Whether to breast- or bottle-feed is a personal and emotional decision and one that you need to feel completely happy about. Before you make up your mind talk it over with your partner and your doctor, and get some first-hand experiences from other mothers.

BREASTFEEDING
Breast milk is the best possible food for your baby because it contains everything he or she needs in the right proportions, and it changes as the baby grows. It contains antibodies which will help protect the baby and it is easily digestible so less likely to cause stomach upsets. Breast-fed babies are also less likely to develop conditions such as eczema and asthma and are less prone to getting some infections.

Breastfeeding has advantages for you as well. Not only is breast milk free and always on "tap," at the correct temperature, it also releases hormones that encourage the uterus to shrink back to its original size more quickly. It uses up calories too, so it will help you get your figure back.

During pregnancy the skin around your nipples will appear darker and raised sebaceous glands will appear as little bumps in the areola, the dark area surrounding the nipple. As your pregnancy progresses the nipples will grow softer. You can help make them more supple by gently massaging them. Take extra care washing and drying your breasts toward the end of pregnancy when they may leak a little, and avoid using soaps that have a drying effect on the skin. You may find that you need to use breast pads to prevent your clothes from getting stained.

Breast milk is free so the only additional cost involved at first is for nursing bras and breast pads. Choose cotton, front-opening nursing bras, with adjustable straps and fastenings because the size of your breasts will change. Wait until after your 30th week of pregnancy before buying a nursing bra – one that fits you then should fit you after the baby is born.

If you want to be able to express

Breastfeeding is the best way to nourish your baby, but bottle feeding with formula can be gradually introduced as he gets older, and can be given by both partners.

milk you will also need a couple of bottles and nipples, sterilizing equipment, and possibly a breast pump.

BOTTLE-FEEDING

Formula has been specially produced for bottle-fed babies. It contains the right balance of vitamins and minerals that a baby needs to thrive. Formula has more protein than breast milk, which means that it takes longer to digest. There are a number of brands to choose from and most are based on cows' milk, although alternatives are available that are designed for children who require special diets for medical reasons. If you use powdered formula, it is very important to follow the instructions because too much or too little can be harmful. The baby will gradually settle into a routine but until then you will need to respond to his or her hunger just as you would if you were breastfeeding.

One of the main advantages of bottle-feeding is that you and your partner can share the feeding between you, so that you can both use the time when you are feeding to get to know your baby.

Hygiene is very important when you bottle-feed because your baby is not getting protection from the antibodies that he or she would have from breast milk. You will need to take particular care in washing and sterilizing bottles and nipples. There are several ways of sterilizing feeding equipment and it is important to choose the method that best suits your needs.

As well as formula you will need at least six bottles and nipples, with caps, a sterilizing unit or container, a bottle brush, and you may also find that a bottle warmer is useful for the night feeding.

Breastfeeding can help you bond with your baby, and the milk will give her everything she needs, including protection against infection.

Massaging your nipples in pregnancy will make them more supple for breastfeeding.

Your growing baby

The fetal brain cells continue to develop and become more sophisticated and the bone centers are beginning to harden. The fetus actively practices breathing, inhaling and exhaling amniotic fluid, as more air sacs develop in the lungs. When too much amniotic fluid is swallowed, you may feel a hiccup. The fetus is now about 13½ in long and now weighs around 1¼ lb.

WEEK 26: CHILDBIRTH CLASSES

You should be about to start childbirth classes. You may choose one or more of these. Childbirth classes show you practical techniques such as relaxation, breathing, and postures for labor and birth. The teacher can answer any questions you may have during the last few months of your pregnancy and will be able to give you information on the birth. Your partner will be welcome at most classes and you will find that they are a good way of meeting other pregnant women and sharing mutual anxieties. Childbirth classes also allow you to feel more in control of a process that can otherwise seem rather daunting.

WHAT THE CLASSES TEACH

Today, most childbirth classes teach a series of techniques gleaned from a number of different approaches, including the Lamaze and Bradley methods, though both Lamaze and Bradley practitioners continue to offer courses in their own specific disciplines. Lamaze classes emphasize the teaching of certain positive responses to the stresses of labor and

You and your body

If you are working you need to decide the date when you are going to stop and inform your employers. Though many women continue working virtually up until the delivery is due, others find that time off before the birth is practical and restorative. If you haven't started taking regular exercise you should do so now, because this will help prepare your body for the rigors of labor.

delivery, including the use of panting and patterned breathing; the Bradley method, on the other hand, stresses more natural breathing methods, as well as the efficacy of good diet and regular exercise.

In almost all classes, you will learn about the stages of labor and will be

Active birth classes

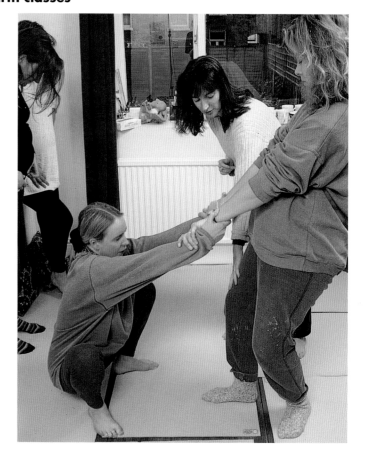

taught appropriate responses in each phase. You will probably learn relaxation techniques to calm you before and during labor, and your partner will almost certainly be expected to act as a full and caring participant during labor. (If your partner is leery of participating, you can usually choose another person to act as your support.)

In addition, most childbirth classes will give you information about the various methods of pain relief that are available, medical and otherwise, and should also arm you with sufficient information so that you can make an educated decision when the time comes.

When choosing a class, speak to your doctor or midwife, as well as to friends who've already gone through the process of childbirth education. If at all possible, make sure that the classes are small and personal. Do ask to sit in on a class before making a final commitment so that you see what is involved.

BREATHING TECHNIQUES

Controlled breathing is important during labor and you need to practice the breathing exercises you will be taught at your classes. In general, breathing needs to be slow and smooth with deep breaths, inhaled through your nose and exhaled through your mouth. A long slow breath at the beginning of each contraction will help oxygenate your blood and this may help relieve any pain caused by the lack of oxygen to the muscles of your uterus. Oxygen is also carried in the blood flowing through the placenta into the umbilical cord, so if you do not get enough, your baby will suffer a shortage too.

During contractions you will be concentrating on each outward breath as this will help you to relax your muscles. It will be important not to over-breathe during the second stage of labor, because this may make you feel dizzy and lightheaded.

If you do find yourself needing to breathe more quickly then you should concentrate on making each breath as light as possible.

Your growing baby

Although still appearing rather scrawny, the fetus is beginning to accumulate fat under the skin. This fat will help regulate body temperature now and after the birth. The fetus is around 13¾ in long and weighs approximately 1½ lb.

Gentle yoga-based exercises are ideal preparation for labor and help you to get ready physically and emotionally, so that you are in tune with the demands on your body. They should always be done under qualified supervision. Exercises include going down into a squatting position (far left and left) in anticipation of labor; massage, which particularly helps if you've got sciatica (below left), and stretching to ease pressure at the base of the spine (below right).

T H E   T H I R D   T R I M E S T E R

WEEK 27: CHOICES IN CHILDBIRTH

Now that you have entered the third trimester you should start planning the kind of birth that you want. If you are having a hospital birth, you will need to discover what facilities are available and then try to plan the birth around them. Although nowadays hospitals do try to accommodate a mother's wishes, not all are able to offer every type of birth. If you want an active or water birth, you will have to find out whether it is possible to arrange at your hospital. If you are having a home birth then having an active birth is easier to arrange. However, you need to remember that if any complications do occur during labor any decisions that you make now may have to be changed to suit the circumstances.

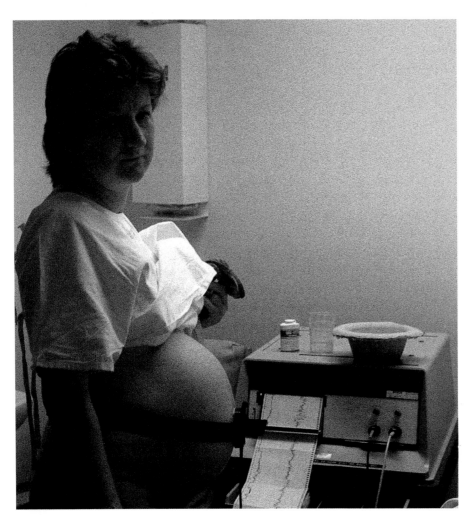

When you give birth in a hospital, special straps might well be put around your belly to attach you to a monitor that checks the strength of your baby's heartbeat.

You and your body

You will be getting noticeably larger and will have put on weight around your chest as well as your breasts. Make sure that you are wearing the correct size of maternity bra. Avoid lying on your back too much because this may make you feel faint, as the enlarged uterus presses directly against blood vessels.

NATURAL CHILDBIRTH

This is when you go through labor and birth without any of the medical procedures that often alter the natural rhythm of labor. Natural childbirth involves the use of breathing and relaxation techniques and sometimes homeopathic remedies.

WATER BIRTH

More popular in Europe than in the U.S., water birth involves spending part of your time in a birth pool, filled with warm water, and giving birth either outside the pool or in the water. The warm water eases contractions, and helps you to relax. Although there is no evidence to prove an increased risk of complications if you have your baby in the water, you should still talk to your doctor before planning to do this.

ACTIVE BIRTH

This means that you are free to move and walk about during labor. Keeping mobile allows the contractions to be more effective. Being in an upright position helps the baby's circulation and encourages the baby to rotate into the best position for

In a natural birth you go through labor without painkillers, using only relaxation methods and maybe homeopathic treatments.

delivery. Gravity aids the baby's descent, and giving birth in a squatting or kneeling position increases the size of the pelvic outlet.

HIGH-TECH BIRTH
Labor is controlled by medical methods such as induction, where labor is started artificially using chemical substances, or the waters are broken manually. Painkilling drugs are used

and an epidural or spinal block to deaden pain may be administered. Epidurals, because of their general safety, are also used increasingly during childbirth.

CAESAREAN BIRTH
This is when the baby is delivered through an incision that is made through the wall of the abdomen into the uterus. It is done under a

general anaesthetic, or sometimes with an epidural or spinal block. If an epidural or spinal block is used you will be awake during the delivery, although a screen is placed across your body so that you don't actually see what is happening. You will be given your baby to hold as soon as it is born. After the birth, the incisions are stitched and you will be kept in hospital for about five days. A Caesarean may be chosen if the reasons that make it necessary are evident before labor begins. This is known as an elective Caesarean. If it is decided on after labor has started, it is known as an emergency Caesarean. Reasons for a Caesarean include abnormal presentation of the baby (that is, not head-first toward the cervix), fetal distress where the baby suffers from lack of oxygen, and a high blood pressure condition in the mother.

When you hold your newborn baby in your arms all the hard work of labor will seem worthwhile.

Your growing baby
The fetus's eyes are open and it will be able to see light through the skin of your abdomen. It will have started to practice sucking and may even be able to suck its thumb or fist. The fetus is now about 14¼ in long and weighs about 1¾ lb.

An active birth involves moving around in labor and adapting different positions that will help your baby's descent.

WEEK 28: THE BIRTHPLAN

You may find it useful to draw up a birthplan – a written set of instructions for your doctor or midwife outlining what procedures you prefer – and which you would like to avoid. Even if there are still things concerning labor or the birth about which you are undecided, writing out a plan will help you focus on the type of birth you want. It will also give you the opportunity to discuss the birth in detail with your partner.

When drawing up your birthplan it is important to remember that there is no right or wrong way to give birth. Your plan should reflect what you feel is right for you, while taking into account your medical history as well as the facilities available at the place where you are going to have your baby.

A birthplan is a guide to how you would like things to be, but in the event of a problem this ideal may become totally impractical so you will need to be flexible. Once you have finalized your birthplan ask for a copy to be kept with your notes so that the doctor or midwife who attend you during labor have it on hand when necessary. You should also keep a copy for yourself so that

You and your body

Your breasts are producing colostrum, the fluid which precedes breast milk. If your breasts are leaking put breast pads or folded tissues inside your bra. If you have a prenatal appointment you will probably have a second blood test to check for anemia. If you are anemic, iron supplements may be offered.

your birth partner can refer to it when he wants to.

BIRTH PARTNER

Although your partner will be encouraged to be with you during labor, you may prefer to have another woman as your actual birth partner, especially if your partner is worried that he may not be able to cope

Write a birthplan with your choices.

Birthplan checklist

The following questions will help you prepare your own birthplan.
- Whom do you wish to have with you during labor – your partner, your mother, a friend? You can choose more than one birth partner.
- Can your birth partner remain with you if you have to have a Caesarean or forceps delivery?
- Do you want to be free to move around during labor, or would you rather be constantly monitored while staying in bed?
- Are there special facilities such as a birthing pool or bean bags available to you?
- Is there any special position you want to use for the birth?
- Do you wish to wear your own clothes during labor and the birth?
- Would you like music, soft lighting, massage or other therapies to help you

cope with getting through labor?
- How do you feel about pain relief? If you want to manage without any, you will need to make sure that everyone knows. If you want pain relief which sort do you want?
- Are you prepared to have an episiotomy if it is required, or would you rather tear naturally?
- Do you want your baby placed straight onto your abdomen or do you want him or her cleaned up first?
- Are you going to breast-feed? If so, do you want to put your baby to the breast immediately?
- Do you want an injection to help deliver the placenta or would you prefer to wait for it to be delivered naturally after the birth?
- How soon after the birth would you like to go home, assuming that there are no complications?

Once you've made your birthplan and put your feelings about your baby's birth in writing, you will feel happier.

with seeing you in pain. Whatever you finally decide, make sure that you talk about it together so that there are no misunderstandings later and so that you don't get upset about the final choice.

Your growing baby

Now fully formed, the fetus would be viable if it were born at 28 weeks, although the body systems are still very immature. The heart is beating at a rate of around 150 beats a minute. The fetus weighs around 2 lb.

If your partner is worried about being with you during a long or painful labor, talk it through with him and make your feelings known if you're counting on his support.

WEEK 29: SPECIAL CARE

If you suffer from a medical condition or blood disorder your pregnancy will require careful managing. Your doctor will need to monitor your progress and you may have to have special prenatal checks. If there is a possible problem, you may be offered another ultrasound during the last trimester, which will clearly show the fetus's breathing movements, how it is lying, and the position of the placenta.

Anemia is caused by an abnormally low level of iron in your red blood cells and is treated with iron supplements. You can build up your body's store of iron by eating a diet which includes red meat, whole grains, dark green leafy vegetables, nuts, and legumes. Liver is not recommended because of the high levels of vitamin A, which could be toxic. A second blood test is done in late pregnancy to check for anemia.

Kidney infection is usually caused by bacterial infection and you should contact your doctor if you think you have a kidney infection. Symptoms are pain, frequent urination accompanied by a burning sensation, and occasionally blood in the urine. Other symptoms you may experience include back pain, high fever, chills, nausea, and vomiting.

You and your body

You will probably be able to feel the fetus's buttocks and feet as it moves around. The fetus will be putting pressure on your stomach and diaphragm now and you will need to sit down and rest more often.

Placenta previa is a rare condition which usually occurs when a woman has had more than one child. The placenta is situated low in the uterus so that it blocks, or partially blocks, the cervix. The pressure of the fetus on the placenta may cause painless bleeding any time after 28 weeks. If this happens, you may have to stay in the hospital until after your baby is born. If the obstruction is particularly severe, your baby may need to be delivered by Caesarean.

As your baby starts to put pressure on your stomach, you'll need to lie down more often to rest.

If the weather is pleasant, you might well prefer to take your regular rests in the garden, but remember to support your legs.

Abruptio placentae is when part of the placenta comes away from the wall of the uterus causing some abdominal pain and bleeding. You should call the doctor immediately. The fetus could be at risk if a large part of the placenta has separated, because it will be deprived of necessary oxygen and nutrients. Sometimes a blood transfusion is necessary and in late pregnancy the baby may be delivered by Caesarean. If only a small part of the placenta has separated, you will need to have complete bedrest until the bleeding has stopped.

Placental insufficiency occurs when the placenta doesn't function efficiently and the fetus grows more slowly than normal because of lack of nourishment. If this happens, you will be told to rest so that the blood flow from the placenta to the fetus can improve. A urine test will also be taken to see whether the health of the fetus is being affected and whether induction is going to be necessary for the birth.

Your growing baby

The fetus is filling almost all the space in your uterus and its head is now more or less in proportion with the rest of the body. The eyebrows and eyelashes are now fully grown and the fetus has quite a lot of hair which is still growing. The eyes, which can now open and close, are beginning to be able to focus properly. The fetus weighs around 2¼ lb and is about 15 in long.

WEEK 30: TRAVEL/BACKACHE

There is no reason why you shouldn't travel during pregnancy, but during the later stages you should check with your doctor if you are going abroad. Airlines may not be willing to take you once you are past 28 weeks because of the risk of a premature labor occurring.

If you want to fly you will need to check with the airline before you buy a ticket; the airline may insist on a medical certificate stating that it is safe for you to travel. If you wish to visit a country where immunization is required, you will have to get medical advice because some vaccines should be avoided completely during pregnancy.

You will probably want to avoid long car journeys toward the end of pregnancy because you may find them uncomfortable. When traveling by car it is important to wear your seatbelt so that it fits neatly across your thighs and above your abdomen, but not across the middle. If the belt was worn across your body it could possibly cause damage to your baby if you were involved in a car accident.

BACKACHE

This can be particularly troublesome during the last months of pregnancy. Hormones have softened your ligaments and the additional weight you are carrying inevitably puts a strain on your stomach muscles, which in turn puts strain on your back muscles. If the backache you are suffering is particularly severe, always check with your doctor because backache can indicate the presence of a kidney infection.

You and your body

You will feel larger and clumsier now and your movements will be slower. It is important to try to maintain good posture to prevent backache. You may have problems sleeping and become a bit breathless if you walk too fast or climb stairs.

Ease upper backache by lying flat on a firm surface with pillows under your head and knees. Lower backache can be helped by kneeling on all fours, with your back straight and your hands and knees well apart, then dropping your head and arching your back. Repeat this exercise several times.

You can help to avoid backache by wearing low-heeled shoes and trying not to hollow your back when you are standing. When you sit down, put a cushion in the small of your back; when you get out of a chair, push yourself right to the edge before attempting to stand up.

A firm mattress will help when you are lying down; when you get up from the lying position, roll over onto your side and then push yourself slowly up. If you have to bend down, always bend your body from the knees and then squat down to pick up anything from the floor.

Your growing baby

The fetus is beginning to move about less vigorously now because it has less space to move around in the uterus. To get comfortable it is likely to adopt a curled-up position with arms and legs crossed. The fetus is now about 15½ in long and weighs around 2½ lb.

Don't fasten your seatbelt over your belly as your baby could be damaged in a accident.

Fasten your seatbelt under your belly and across your thighs to protect your baby.

Bending in pregnancy

1 *In later pregnancy particularly, bend your knees, not from the waist, and pick up the object when you are squatting.*

2 *As you get up from the squatting position, keep your back straight and lift up the object at arm's length.*

3 *As you gradually become upright, straighten your bent knees without making any jerky movements.*

How to relieve backache

1 *To relieve painful aches in your lower back in pregnancy, try this exercise. Kneel down on the floor on all fours with your back straight, your head facing down, and your hands and knees spaced well apart.*

2 *Drop your head right down and arch your back to stretch out the painful muscles, hold for several seconds, then release, raising your head again. Repeat the exercise several times for the best relief.*

WEEK 31: DEALING WITH DISCOMFORT

You and your body

Breathlessness may be more of a problem now, especially if you overdo things. Try to get as much rest as possible and slow down any exercise regimen to a pace that suits you. If your breasts feel uncomfortable when you go to bed, wear a maternity or specially designed sleep bra at night.

The fetus is getting quite big and will be putting pressure on your diaphragm, which may mean that you are now finding it more difficult to breathe. This breathlessness should pass once the fetus's head drops into the pelvis and becomes engaged in a few weeks' time. Try sitting and standing as straight as possible, and put some extra pillows behind your shoulders when you are in bed.

You are likely to need a larger size bra toward the end of pregnancy and the one that you buy now should fit you after the baby is born. If you are intending to breastfeed, buy a front-opening nursing bra that will be suitable to wear both now and after the birth.

Choose a bra with wide adjustable straps and fastenings and that has a broad supportive band under the cups. Make sure that the cups fit comfortably and do not gape under the arms. Buy one made from cotton or a cotton blend that will be more comfortable to wear, and allow your skin to breathe properly, particularly in hot weather.

BRAXTON HICKS CONTRACTIONS
During pregnancy you will experience contractions that may be uncomfortable but are not usually painful. These are known as Braxton Hicks contractions, which tighten the muscles of the uterus about every 20 minutes throughout pregnancy, although you have probably not been aware of them during the early months. In the last weeks of

pregnancy these contractions become more noticeable as they begin to prepare the uterus for labor by drawing up the cervix and making it thinner. When you have these

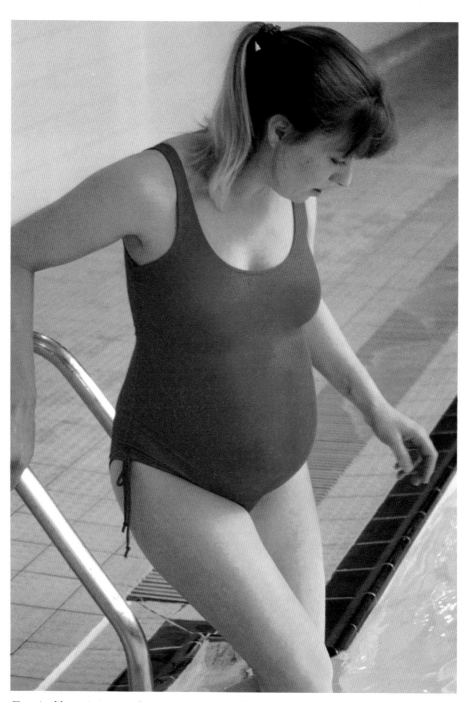

Exercise like swimming, where you are supported in the water, will keep you fit in late pregnancy. It will also relieve backache as the swimming motion will stretch the back muscles.

contractions, practice your breathing techniques for labor.

KICK COUNTS

You can check on your baby's well-being by keeping a count of the fetal movements. If there is any concern about the fetus's development you may be asked to keep a kick chart recording the first 10 movements each day. For your own peace of mind you should be aware of these movements so that if for any reason they become less frequent, or even stop altogether, you will notice immediately. If you are ever concerned about lack of movement, seek some medical advice immediately because it could indicate some trouble with the fetus.

As your pregnancy progresses and the fetus gets bigger it has less room to maneuver, so movements will be more noticeable, but less frequent. By the end of your pregnancy the fetus will probably move between 10 and 12 times in a 12-hour period.

Keep a kick count of your baby's movements on a chart, so that you can monitor any noticeable changes and seek medical help if you feel it is necessary.

Try sitting in a yoga position with your back straight to alleviate the pressure your baby is putting on your diaphragm.

Your growing baby

The organs are almost completely developed, apart from the lungs which are still not fully mature. The brain is still growing and the nerve cells and connections are now working. A protective sheath is developing around the nerve fibers so that messages travel faster, enabling the fetus to learn more. It can feel pain and will move if prodded and you can feel it jump at loud noises. The fetus is around 15¾ in long and weighs about 3 lb.

WEEK 32: POSITIONS FOR LABOR

It is a good idea to practice some of the positions that will help you through the different stages of labor. During the first stage you should try to stay upright and keep active. Being upright will make your contractions stronger and more efficient. It will also allow gravity to keep the baby's head pressed down, which will help your cervix to dilate faster so that labor is speeded up. Remaining active will give you more control over labor so that you should feel less pain. If you are lying down, your uterus presses on the large blood vessels running down your back and this can reduce the blood flow through the placenta to and from the baby. If you feel you want to lie down during labor, try to position yourself on your side rather than on your back.

COPING WITH CONTRACTIONS

You should aim to give the fetus as much room as possible in your pelvis and the best way to achieve this is by keeping your knees well apart and leaning forward so that the uterus tilts away from your spine. During the first-stage contractions it may help to lean against your partner, or if you prefer you can kneel down resting your arms and head on a cushion on the seat of a chair. If you find being upright tiring, try kneeling on all fours. This allows you to keep the weight of the fetus off your lower back. By the time your contractions are coming every few minutes you may want to adopt a squatting position, or you could try kneeling forward onto a pile of cushions or a bean bag with your legs wide apart. It may help if your

You and your body

If you work, you may have left by now or will have a date when you are going to leave. Enjoy the last weeks of your pregnancy and spend time singing and talking to your baby. You may find the fetal movements uncomfortable now that it is so much bigger. Occasionally, you may feel its feet getting stuck under your ribs.

partner massages your back while you are in this position.

When you reach the second stage you'll want to find a comfortable position for the birth. If you lie on your back you will literally have to push the baby uphill. If you remain upright your abdominal muscles will work more efficiently as you bear down, and gravity will help the baby out. Try squatting, supported on both sides, or with your partner supporting you from behind, so that your pelvis is at its widest and you have control over the pelvic floor

Labor positions

1 *Relax on all fours by flopping forward onto a pile of cushions or a bean bag to give the fetus as much room as possible in the pelvis. Your partner can help by massaging your back.*

2 *Take the weight of the baby off your spine by kneeling on the floor on all fours with your arms and legs wide apart. Keep the small of your back flat and not hollowed.*

Your growing baby

The fetus is now very energetic and it will have periods of extreme activity, and you will feel it twisting and turning. As it continues to grow it will have less and less room to move in, so it will soon settle, probably in the head-down position, ready for birth. The fetus measures about 16 in and weighs about 3½ lb.

which you will need to relax. Kneeling with your legs wide apart and supported on both sides is another good position for pushing.

Once you have tried these positions, experiment with others that you feel may be right for you during labor. Try them on the floor, on the bed, leaning on or against furniture, or using your partner for support. This way, when you are in labor, you will already know how to get into positions that are comfortable for you and that will help you cope with contractions.

Partner support

1 *Practice using your partner for support during labor by leaning back against him, allowing him to take your weight.*

2 *Stand with feet well apart and lean on your partner, putting your head on your arms to ease pressure on your uterus.*

3 *Kneel on all fours with your forearms on the floor and your knees spread wide so that your abdomen is hanging between them. It can help to rock backward and forward in this position.*

4 *In this squatting position, your pelvis is wide open and the baby's head is pressed down. You may find that it helps to place your hands on the floor to give yourself some support.*

WEEK 33: EMOTIONS IN LATE PREGNANCY

It is not just your body that is going through great changes while you are pregnant. Your whole way of life is changing and this can lead to conflicting emotions, especially during the last few months. You may wonder how you are going to cope with all the new responsibilities and be concerned about your baby – whether it will be born perfect in every way. Vivid dreams are common at this time and can be upsetting, especially if they are about the birth or babies. You may even feel occasionally that the whole thing has been a ghastly mistake and that you want to go back to the way things were before you became pregnant. Don't worry, all these feelings are quite normal.

It helps to talk about your fears and concerns, either to your partner or to a close friend who has had similar feelings. Childbirth classes are also a good place to discuss these worries, especially as you will be with other women who are experiencing the same emotions. If you find that talking about it doesn't help and that anxiety is taking over your life, discuss how you feel with your midwife or doctor.

YOUR PARTNER

It is easy to forget that an expectant father is also going through emotional changes as he comes to terms with impending parenthood. He doesn't have any outward sign of the change that is about to occur in his life, but that doesn't mean he isn't feeling the same concerns as you. He also has additional worries about you and how you will cope during labor; he may even secretly fear for your safety during the birth. If he is now solely responsible for providing financially for you and the baby he

You and your body

Your weight gain should have slowed down. If it hasn't and you are still gaining more than 2¼ lb a week, you should check with your doctor that everything is all right.

may be feeling considerable stress.

Make time to talk to each other about your feelings and try to ensure that these last weeks before the birth are special for you both. Share the preparation for the birth so that each of you is involved in what is going to happen. Plan some treats where you can be alone together, such as a special dinner at a favorite restaurant, a trip to the theater, or a weekend away at a hotel. By making time for yourselves you are less likely to have misunderstandings that could lead to hurt and disappointment.

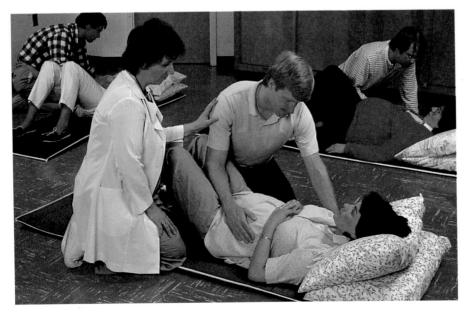

At childbirth classes you learn what to expect in labor and the different positions you can adopt. Your partner is usually expected to come with you and find out how he can help.

Your growing baby

The fingernails are fully formed although the toenails are not quite so advanced. The vernix covering the skin has become thicker. The lungs are almost fully developed and the fetus will be practicing breathing in preparation for the birth. It measures around 16½ in and now weighs about 4 lb.

OTHER CHILDREN

If you have other children you may have told them about the new baby early on in your pregnancy. Very young children will need to have it explained to them over and over again, because the concept of a new baby is hard for them to grasp. Older children will probably be very excited and will enjoy being involved in any preparations you are making for their brother or sister.

How children react once the baby has arrived depends a lot on their age and personality, as well as their relationship with you. A preschool child may react by misbehaving for a period in an attempt to get your attention. A toddler, who has recently been potty trained, may start wetting or soiling him- or herself again. Both age groups may start waking at night. Use common sense and tact to minimize any problems. Talk to your children about the new baby, encourage their help and involvement when he or she has been born but always make sure that they have time with you on their own.

Let an older child feel your belly, and talk to him or her about their new brother or sister, so they can get used to the idea of a new family member.

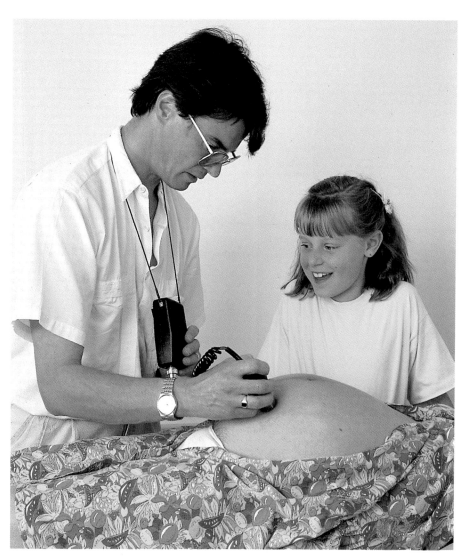

When your doctor checks your baby's heartbeat, let any older children be present if they are interested.

WEEK 34: OLDER FIRST-TIME MOTHERS

If you are 35 or over, you will probably have been offered an amniocentesis because of the higher risk of fetal abnormality. The amniotic fluid will have been screened for a number of chromosomal disorders, which include Down's syndrome and spina bifida. Of course, you are not obliged to have this test, but many mothers prefer to do so because they find it reassuring.

It is important that you attend all your prenatal checkups so that a close check can be kept on you and the unborn baby all through the pregnancy. The risk to the baby during labor and birth does increase somewhat with rising maternal age, but many different factors affect labor, including the general health of the mother during pregnancy. Although nearly 70 percent of women over 30 have normal deliveries, there is a slightly greater risk of complications during labor for women who are over the age of 35. On the other hand, because older mothers tend to have a higher socioeconomic status and more education than younger mothers, their prenatal care is generally better.

BIRTH AND THE OLDER MOTHER
Most older women go full term, and if you are between 30 and 34 there is no reason why you shouldn't have a natural birth. If you are 35 or over, or if there is a suggestion that your baby may be small, you may have to have continuous monitoring. This may also be necessary if there is a likelihood of a prolonged labor, or if the waters, when they break, show some sign of staining. This means that you will be unable to move around freely. But this is a very small price to pay for having a normal, healthy baby.

You and your body

Your blood pressure may be slightly elevated and you will probably be told to take things easy. Swelling of the hands and feet could also be a problem so get as much rest as possible, preferably with your feet up.

Seeing her baby on an ultrasound scan can be very reassuring for an older mother.

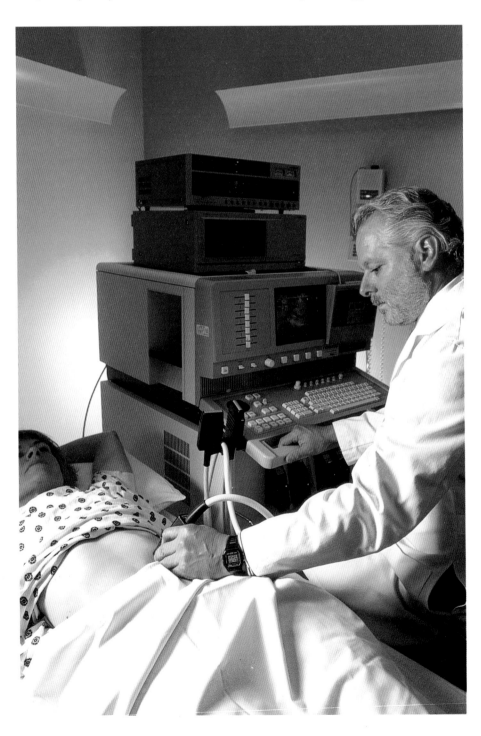

Babies born to older mothers have a slightly greater chance of being born preterm. This is sometimes because of the failure of the placenta, which means the baby is no longer getting sufficient oxygen and nourishment. If this happens you may have to have a labor induced delivery, or you may be offered a Caesarean section.

Your growing baby

The weight gain continues to increase. The eyes respond to bright lights and the fetus will start to practice blinking; eyebrows and eyelashes are fully developed. A boy's testicles will have descended into the groin. The fetus is 17 in long and now weighs about 4½ lb.

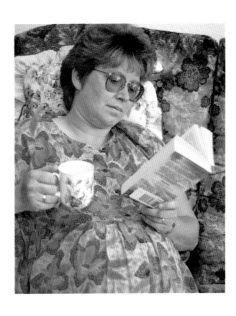

Below: The doctor will talk about your baby and may give you a printout of your scan.

Right: As time progresses, you will find you need more rest with your back supported.

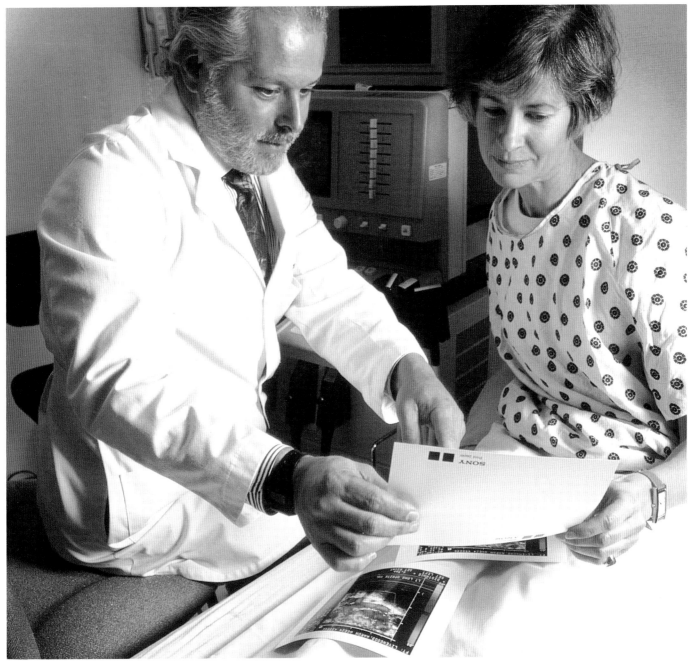

WEEK 35: FINAL PREPARATIONS

Even though your baby is not due for some weeks, you should be ready in case he or she decides to put in an early appearance. Check the baby's room and make sure all the sheets and blankets have been washed and aired. Sort out all the baby clothes and put the ones you will want immediately after the birth in your hospital bag.

It's a good idea to stock up on nonperishable goods and to fill the freezer. This will save you from having to do a lot of shopping over the next few weeks and will allow you more time with the baby when you first come home.

Make sure you know where your partner is going to be over the next few weeks; if he is out and about you may want to consider renting a beeper so that you can keep in constant touch. Keep your car filled with gas and make sure that you both know the quickest route to the hospital. Have a list of emergency numbers, including a local taxi firm, beside the telephone.

THE HOSPITAL

Pack what you want to take to the hospital several weeks before the delivery date; keep the bag where you can easily get it when the time comes. Remember that there are three separate aspects to consider: labor, your hospital stay, and going-home clothes for you and the baby.

You should bring any personal items that will make life more comfortable for you during labor. Include anything from a cassette

You and your body

Discuss any worries you may have about labor and birth with your doctor or midwife. You will be feeling tired and even a little fed up, so try to get as much rest as you can. Pay special attention to your diet: you will be needing another 200 calories a day during these last weeks. Some practical planning now can save time and forestall anxiety at the time of labor and delivery.

player and your favorite music to a washcloth and massage oils. You might want to pack a deck of cards or even a bottle of champagne (check with your doctor on this). Leave some room for last-minute items such as an ice pack for backache and even a snack and drink for your partner. Don't forget to put your birthplan right at the top so that you can give this to the doctor when you arrive at the hospital. It is

It is a good idea to buy vegetables and other food that can be cooked and frozen in preparation for when you return from the hospital.

sensible to pack things for labor separately, since you will want to be able to get to them quickly.

How much you pack for the hospital depends on your planned length of stay after the birth. The hospital may issue a list of the items that you will need to bring with you. But if it doesn't, ask your doctor or midwife whether you need to take in baby clothes and diapers, or contact the maternity unit direct. If aren't too tired, you might want to write cards to your friends and relatives announcing your baby's arrival, so remember to include birth announcement cards, your address book, and stamps. You may also want to bring along a camera or possibly a camcorder to take photographs or a film of your baby.

You will need clothes for you and the baby when it's time for you to return home. It is sensible to pack a small bag now with all the items you think you'll want for your return journey; you can either bring it with you or your partner can bring it later. Remember that although you will feel considerably slimmer than you were before the birth, it takes quite a while before you get your figure back, so your going-home outfit will still need to be loose and comfortable to wear.

You might need to get to the hospital quickly, so have your bag packed and keep a local taxi number close by.

It is sensible to pack a small bag for your brief stay in the hospital well in advance in case you have to leave in a rush. Don't forget some clothes for your new baby to wear.

Your growing baby

The fetus is putting on weight each day and now fills most of the uterus, so you may find it uncomfortable when it starts to move around. The fetus now does body rolls rather than the more energetic movements it was able to make when it was smaller. It is now about 17½ in long and weighs around 5 lb.

WEEK 36: DISCOMFORTS IN LATE PREGNANCY

You and your body

You will be able to feel the top of your uterus just below your breastbone. This can make breathing uncomfortable and you may suffer from pain in your ribcage. Your prenatal checks will be weekly from now on.

As you find getting around more difficult and everything generally more of an effort, you may become irritable over the smallest things. You will be impatient for your baby to arrive, and concern about the impending birth and worries about how you will cope with being a parent can make you short-tempered, especially with your partner. Tell him how you are feeling so that he understands why you are being so irritable and perhaps not giving him as much attention as usual.

Aches or pains around your pubic area, in your groin, or down the inside of your legs can be caused by your baby's head pressing on the nerves, or by your pelvic joints beginning to soften in preparation for labor. Pain under your ribs is caused by the expanding uterus pushing the ribs up. These aches and pains are not serious, but they can be quite uncomfortable. Sitting or standing as straight as you can, or stretching upward, will help ease most of these discomforts, although

you may find lying down better for relief of pelvic pain. If you get severe pain in your abdomen, or if you suffer any abdominal pain that is also accompanied by vaginal bleeding, you must get in touch with your doctor at once.

It is quite common to suffer from heartburn and nausea toward the end of pregnancy. This is caused by the enlarged uterus pressing on your stomach. It often helps to eat small

Soaking in a warm bath can help to relieve any aches and pains you are suffering.

meals at frequent intervals, rather than two or three big meals a day.

PRENATAL CHECK-UP
An internal examination may be carried out to check the size of your pelvis. If there is any concern about the size of your pelvis in relation to your baby's size, or there is some other reason for the baby's delivery not being straightforward, a Caesarean may be discussed. If this is thought to be necessary, the doctor at the hospital where the delivery is to take place will explain the medical procedures that will be used.

As your baby increases in size, you may begin to find breathing uncomfortable and get some pain in your ribcage.

Your growing baby

The nervous system is maturing and the fetus is getting ready for birth by starting to practise breathing movements, sucking, and swallowing. It is now about 18¼ in long and weighs around 5½ lb.

In this late stage of pregnancy you will probably be able to feel the top of your uterus which is now positioned just below your breastbone.

WEEK 37: AS BIRTH APPROACHES

Your growing baby

The lanugo, the fine hair that covers the fetus's body, is beginning to wear off. The fetus has started to produce a hormone called cortisone which will help the lungs to become fully matured so that they are ready to cope with breathing once it is born. The fetus will be practising breathing although there isn't any air in its lungs yet. The fetus is now about 18½ in long and weighs around 6 lb.

Between weeks 36 and 38 the baby's head is likely to "engage." This is when it settles downward, deep in your pelvis ready for the birth. You should feel some relief from the pressure in your abdomen when this happens which is why it is sometimes referred to as "lightening." You will start to feel less breathless now because the baby is no longer putting any pressure on your diaphragm and your lungs.

If this is not your first baby, but your second or third child, the head may not engage until you actually go into labor.

PREMATURE AND TWIN BIRTHS
If the baby is born before 37 weeks it will be described as being preterm or premature. Most premature babies are cared for either in the regular nursery or in a neonatal intensive care unit. Babies are given expert care and attention in these facilities,

This is probably the last time for a while that you will have time to yourself, so make the most of it and rest often.

With modern technology even babies as young as 24 weeks can survive in the neonatal intensive care units.

so that even those that are born as young as 24 weeks have a reasonable chance of survival.

If you are giving birth to twins, the labor doesn't usually take any longer than if you are giving birth to a single baby.

Because twins tend to be smaller babies, the labor and birth can often be easier and less painful to endure. Once the birth canal has been stretched to allow one baby to be born, the second baby will usually be born quite quickly afterward. If twins share the placenta, they will both be born before it is delivered. Even if they are fraternal twins and each has her own placenta they will usually be born first, although occasionally one baby is born, followed by its own placenta, before the second baby arrives.

You and your body

Your baby could arrive at any time from now until the end of week 42, so check that you have everything organized. You will probably be able to visit the hospital about now and see where you are going to give birth. Don't be afraid to ask questions if there is anything you don't understand about hospital procedures.

Sometime between now and the birth, you may experience a sudden burst of energy, known as the nesting instinct. Don't overdo things and decide to spring-clean your whole house. Remember that you will shortly need all your energy reserves for the exhausting demands of labor.

As the birth approaches, it is a good time for you and your partner to start making a list of names that you both like.

WEEK 38: INDUCTION/PAIN RELIEF IN LABOR

You and your body

You will notice that the fetus is moving about less now that it is head down in the uterus. You may be feeling tired and rather depressed about the waiting so try to keep busy.

Sometimes labor has to be started artificially because of a problem such as preeclampsia, bleeding, diabetes, or you are well past your due date and the placenta is no longer working efficiently. Induction involves several techniques:

Artificial rupture of the membranes (ARM) This involves puncturing the amniotic sac in which the baby is sealed so that the increased pressure on the cervix causes the contractions to become much stronger.

Pitocin drip A hormone that stimulates contractions, known as oxytocin or, more commonly, by its trade name Pitocin, is administered – generally by intravenous drip – to help contractions remain constant and steady. This may lead to stronger contractions than you would otherwise have had.

PAIN RELIEF

You will have been told about the various forms of pain relief at childbirth classes. If you want to have a completely natural birth make sure that this is marked clearly on your birthplan and inform the medical staff who will be attending you during labor.

Remember that you can always change your mind later if you find coping with the pain too difficult. If you have decided to opt for some form of pain relief, there are a number of options you can choose from:

Injections Drugs like meperidine hydrochloride (Demerol) can be given during the first stage of labor. They will help you relax and relieve pain but they can affect the baby, making him sleepy at birth.

"Gas and air" (Entonox) A mixture of oxygen and nitrous oxide that is breathed in through a mask and takes the edge off pain. The gas is processed in your lungs so it doesn't affect the baby. This procedure, however, is now becoming increasingly uncommon.

Epidural A local anaesthetic is injected into the space between your spinal column and the spinal cord, numbing the nerves that serve the uterus. It may also numb your leg nerves, making it hard for you to move around the hospital. An epidural may also be used if a Caesarean delivery is performed because it allows the mother to stay awake, but be pain free, while her baby is being delivered.

An anaesthesiologist is needed to give an epidural injection, which takes around 30 minutes to set up, and then usually requires topping up every hour and a half.

Other, less common, blocks may also be administered. These include the pudendal block, which is given in the perineum or around the vagina to ease the pain of delivery, and the spinal or low spinal block, in which the anaesthetic is injected

In the past oxygen and nitrous oxide were given for pain relief during contractions. This method is seldom used today.

straight into the spinal fluid.

Alternative pain relief Both of the alternative therapies – acupuncture and hypnosis – can be used to relieve pain during childbirth, but if

An epidural injection into the spinal area helps deaden the nerves around the uterus.

In Europe, pads from a TENS machine can be put on your back to ease labor pains.

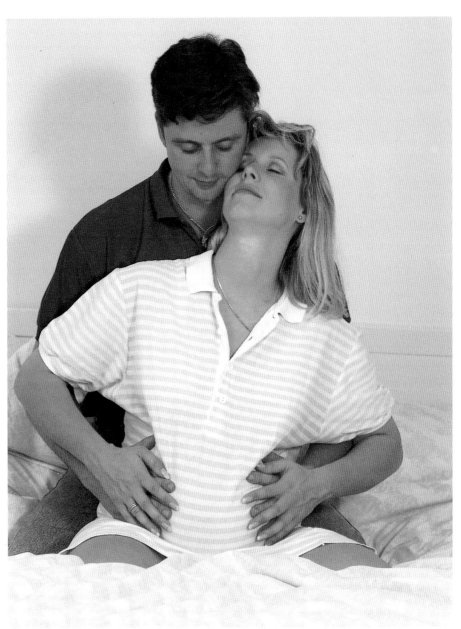

At the most painful times in your labor, lean on your partner for support and encouragement. He can also massage your back if it is really painful.

you are having a hospital birth you will need to get permission so that you can have a private practitioner with you during labor.

Used in the correct way by a professional practitioner, massage, aromatherapy, and reflexology can all help to ease the pain and discomfort experienced in labor. You should get some expert advice from the relevant associations and then talk to your doctor before the birth if you intend to use any of these special techniques during your labor.

Your growing baby

The fetus has put on some fat so that it now appears more rounded and its skin has a pinkish look. The hair may be as long as 2 in and the nails already need cutting. The vernix, which has been protecting the skin of the growing fetus from the amniotic fluid, is beginning to dissolve. At this stage of your pregnancy, the fetus measures about 19 in and weighs around 6½ lb.

WEEK 39: COMPLICATIONS DURING BIRTH

The ideal position for your baby to be born is with its head lying down with its back against your abdomen. This way it has less distance to rotate in the birth canal. Sometimes a baby is in an abnormal position which can make birth more complicated, but this does not necessarily mean that it can't be born in the normal way.

An occipito posterior position means that the baby is lying with its back toward your back and, if it fails to turn, will be delivered normally, but will be born face up. This way of lying often leads to what is known as a "back labor."

In a deep transverse arrest, the baby's head partially rotates in the birth canal and then becomes stuck with its face toward one side. The baby will need to be helped out.

Disproportion means that the baby's head is too big for your pelvis. Rarely, a scan will be done to decide whether there is enough room for a normal delivery to take place. If there isn't, your baby will probably be born by Caesarean.

BREECH BIRTH

A small number of babies don't turn around in the normal way in the last few weeks of pregnancy. This means that their feet or buttocks would be delivered first so the birth canal will not have been stretched sufficiently when the head, the largest part of the baby's body, is then ready to be born.

Doctors have different opinions about the best way of delivering a breech baby; some insist that a Caesarean is the safest method, others believe that birth should take place under an epidural, and some think that if the mother remains mobile throughout the first stage of labor the baby will manage to get itself into a good position for the actual birth. It may then be helped out by using forceps or by the vacuum extraction method.

Birth positions

A normal birth

A breech birth

You and your body

The waiting is nearly over and you will probably be feeling both excited and apprehensive. You may be having quite strong Braxton Hicks contractions as the cervix softens in readiness for the birth. Although you may be feeling heavy and weary, don't simply sit around waiting for something to happen. Keep up your social life and talk to other friends from your childbirth classes who are at the same stage as you.

FORCEPS DELIVERY

In a forceps delivery, your legs will be put up in stirrups and then the forceps, which are like a pair of large, shallow metal spoons, will be inserted into the vagina and cupped around the baby's head. The doctor helps the baby out while you push.

VACUUM EXTRACTION

Vacuum extraction is sometimes used instead of the forceps method. With this technique the doctor places a suction cup on the baby's head and the baby is then sucked out as you push down hard with each contraction.

If the birth canal is not going to be big enough for the baby's head and there is a risk that the perineum may tear, a small cut may be made in this area under local anaesthetic.

Your growing baby

The fetus is now able to function on its own, although it is still getting nourishment from the placenta. The fetus is in position for the impending birth and is now about 19¼ in long and weighs around 7 lb.

This type of incision is called an epi-siotomy and is stitched after the birth, again under local anaesthetic.

FETAL MONITORING

This keeps a check on the unborn baby's heartbeat during labor and birth. Monitoring can be done the low-tech way by simply placing a stethoscope against the patient's abdomen, or through electronic fetal monitoring (EFM).

There are two types of EFM and they both give a continuous readout of the baby's heart and uterine con-tractions; if the EFM method is used then you are having a high-tech birth.

There are two different methods of fetal monitoring. The basic method is to listen to the fetal heartbeat using a fetal stethoscope (top right). The position of the baby will also be checked at the same time (right). Electronic fetal monitoring (EFM) (below) involves placing a belt around your belly which is attached to a monitor. This gives a continuous readout of the baby's heart.

WEEK 40: LABOR AND BIRTH

It is unlikely that you won't recognize the beginnings of labor as the signs, when they come, are generally unmistakable. There are three main indications that labor is about to start, or has started, and they can occur in any order. Once one or more of these has occurred you should let your doctor or midwife know immediately:

A show The protective plug, which sealed the cervix at the neck of the uterus, comes away and passes down the vagina. It usually appears as a small amount of bloodstained mucus. A show occurs before labor starts or during the first stage.

Waters breaking The membranes of the amniotic sac in which your baby has been floating break, causing either a trickle or a sudden gush of clear fluid from the vagina. If the fluid is yellow, greenish, or brown in color you will need to go to the hospital immediately because the baby may be in distress. Your waters can break hours before labor starts or when it is well underway.

Contractions The regular tightening of the muscles of the uterus occurs throughout labor. During the first stage, the contractions thin out and dilate the cervix from closed to 10 cm open; in the second stage they help to push the baby down the vagina and after the birth they then deliver the placenta (afterbirth). For most women they feel rather like bad menstrual cramps. Contractions may be also be accompanied by uncomfortable backache, sickness, and some diarrhea.

Your growing baby

Your baby is lying curled up, head down, in the fetal position with legs drawn up underneath and waiting to be born. He or she now measures about 19¾ in and weighs around 7½ lb.

You and your body

You will probably be impatient for labor to start as you approach your EDD. If nothing has happened by your due date try not to be too disappointed; only around five percent of babies actually arrive on the date they were expected. Keep yourself busy and make plans for each day so that you are not just sitting and waiting for something to happen. Once you are close to your EDD you may feel more confident wearing a sanitary napkin just in case your waters break.

During the first stage of labor, you can involve your partner by leaning and holding onto him for comfort and also physical support.

Your partner can help and encourage you when you're on all fours to keep the weight of the baby off your back in an active birth.

STAGES OF LABOR

The first stage: There are three stages of labor and the first is usually the longest, lasting generally from 12 hours upward for a first baby. Contractions, which may have started off as mild and infrequent will, by the end of the first stage, be very strong and coming close together. Once they are coming regularly

Tips for labor

● Keep active for as long as you can during the first stage of labor.

● Don't be on your own: get your partner, mother or a friend to stay with you once labor has started.

● If your waters break check that the fluid is clear: yellow, greenish, or brown fluid could mean that your baby is in distress and you should go to the hospital immediately.

● Try different positions to help you

cope with the pain of contractions.

● Ask for pain relief if you need it.

● Get your birth partner to make sure your wishes are known to whoever is delivering your baby. You may be too busy coping with contractions to explain clearly what you want.

● Put your baby to the breast soon after the birth. This will stimulate your milk supply and help to speed up the delivery of the placenta.

every 10 minutes, or are each lasting for around 45 seconds, you should start getting ready to go to the hospital, or call the midwife if you are having your baby at home. When you get to the hospital, or the midwife attending you at home arrives, you will be examined to see how far your cervix has dilated and your blood pressure will be checked.

Although you will be able to carry on fairly normally for quite a lot of the first stage you should have someone with you. It is advisable to eat very little once labor has begun in case you need an emergency anaesthetic for any reason and to avoid being sick.

Toward the end of the first stage you will go into what is known as the transitional stage which can last for anything up to an hour. During this transitional period your baby moves down the birth canal and you will feel pressure on your back which may make you want to start pushing, even though the cervix is not fully dilated. By using the breathing techniques you have been taught you will be able to control this urge.

The second stage: Once the cervix is fully dilated and you start pushing the baby out you have entered the second stage. It can last for as little as half an hour or for as long as two hours or more. Once the baby's head is visible to the doctor or midwife she will tell you to start pushing. When the head reaches the vaginal opening you will be told to pant in short breaths so that the head can be delivered as slowly as possible. This allows the skin and muscle of the perineum to stretch so that the head can be born. If tearing seems likely an episiotomy, a small cut in the perineum, the area between the vagina and anus, may be given. Once the head is born your baby's body will follow quickly.

When your baby is delivered it may be lifted onto your stomach for you to see it. The umbilical cord will be clamped and cut and the doctor or midwife will check the baby to make sure that he is all right and breathing properly. You may want to put your baby to the breast, and you'll certainly want to admire him or her with your partner and welcome your child into the world.

With a water birth, still uncommon in the U.S., contractions can be eased by the warm water. Your baby can be delivered in the water or outside.

If you have your baby in the water, he will be given to you immediately after the birth for you and your partner to cuddle.

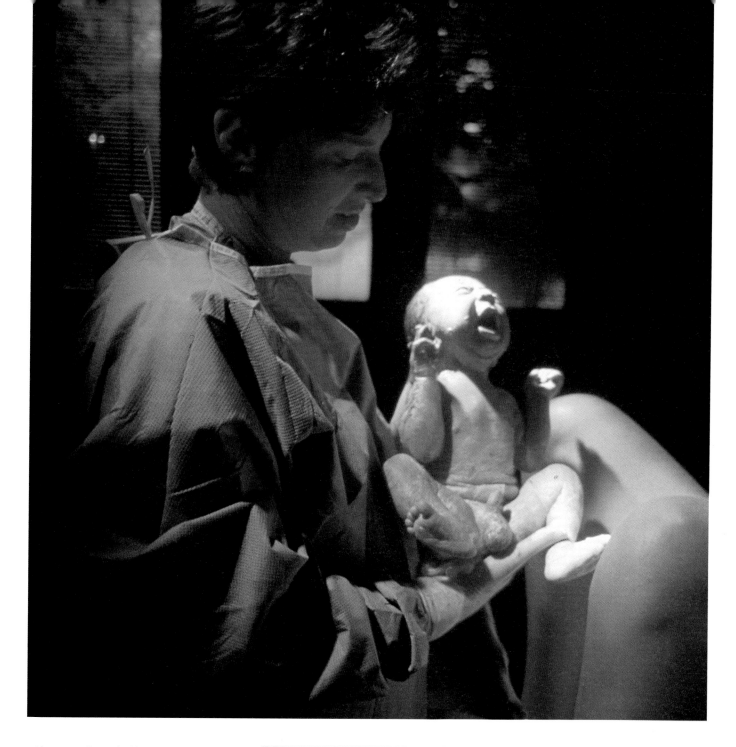

Above: A doctor holding a newborn baby boy, with the umbilical cord still attached, at a home delivery.

Right: With a Caesarean the baby is delivered through an incision. It is performed when there are risks from natural childbirth.

The third stage: The final stage of labor is the birth of the placenta, which usually takes less than half an hour. You may be given an injection to speed up the delivery. The midwife will check to see that the placenta is whole and that nothing has been left inside you. If you have had an episiotomy it will be stitched up.

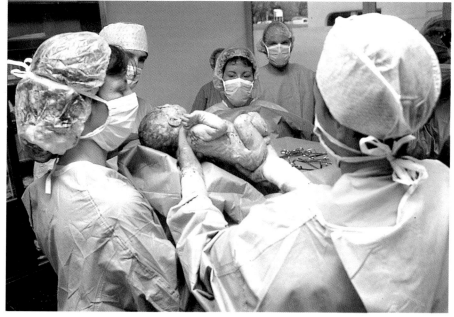

POST-PARTUM CARE

Although your new baby will probably give you intense emotional satisfaction, you may well be physically uncomfortable. Your body has gone through many changes during pregnancy and it will take a while for it to return to its pre-pregnancy state.

Six weeks or so after the birth your doctor will examine you to make sure that everything is returning to normal; this also gives you a chance to discuss any worries you may have. The doctor will take your blood pressure and check a sample of your urine. Your breasts and abdomen will be examined and the doctor will make sure that any stitches have healed properly. You will probably have an internal examination to check the size and position of your uterus and you may have a Pap test if one is due.

If your baby was born in the hospital, a doctor or midwife will probably talk to you about contraception before you go home. Alternatively, you can discuss this at your first check-up. Don't take any risks; to avoid getting pregnant again you

should use contraception as soon as you resume intercourse with your partner. While breastfeeding may prevent conception, it is by no means a dependable safeguard.

If you were not immune to rubella (German measles) during your pregnancy, you may be offered the immunization before you leave the hospital or at your six-week check-up. Ask your doctor if you are at all unsure about your immunity.

YOUR BODY

Immediately after the birth your breasts will produce colostrum, a high-protein liquid full of antibodies. Then, after the pregnancy hormones decline, your main milk supply should come in around the third or fourth day. At this time the breasts swell, feel hard, and can sometimes be painful. Bathing them with warm water is soothing, and letting the baby have frequent feeding will also help. This initial swelling subsides after a few days as both you and your baby get used to feeding. However, if you have decided to bottle-feed,

your breasts will remain full for a few days until they gradually stop producing milk. Your breasts will probably never be quite as firm as they were before pregnancy, but a well-fitting support bra and exercise will help greatly.

After delivery your abdomen will probably be quite flabby and wrinkled because of slack muscles and stretched skin. Gentle post-partum exercises will help tighten up your abdominal and vaginal muscles, so make time to do them every day. If you feel you're not disciplined enough to exercise on your own, consider joining a post-partum class.

Following the birth you will have a vaginal discharge which is known as lochia. This will be like a very heavy period for a few days, with the flow gradually getting lighter until it disappears within a few weeks. Use maternity pads or large sanitary napkins to absorb the discharge because there is a risk of infection if you use tampons in the early weeks after the birth. Your

Your newborn will find your physical presence very reassuring during the first days after the birth. She will also find your smell comfortingly familiar.

Post-partum exercises

Pelvic floor: Lie flat on the floor with your legs drawn up and slightly apart. Close the back passage by drawing it in, hold for the count of four, then relax. Do as often as possible.

Tummy toner: Sit up with knees bent and feet flat on the floor. Fold arms in front. Lean back until you feel the abdominal muscles tighten, hold, then sit up and relax. Repeat several times.

1 *Curl-ups: This exercise will help strengthen your vertical abdominal muscles. Lie on your back with a pillow under your head, your knees bent and your feet flat on the floor.*

2 *Pull in your abdominal muscles and, raising your head, stretch your arms toward your knees. Hold for a count of five and then relax slowly. Repeat several times.*

Leg slide: Lie with your head on a pillow with the small of your back pressed against the floor and your knees bent. Gently slide one leg away from your body until it is fully extended, keeping the small of your back pressed against the floor for as long as you can. Slowly draw the leg back toward your body and then repeat with the other leg. Do this several times.

uterus will take about six weeks to return to its original size. If you are breastfeeding you may feel it contract as you feed the baby.

If your perineum (the skin between the vagina and anus) was bruised during labor, or if you had stitches, you will find that anything that puts pressure on the area painful. Soreness can be soothed with an ice pack (or ice cubes wrapped in a washcloth) held against the perineum or by Sitz baths (ask your doctor). Try drying the area with a hand-held hair dryer, set on

cool, rather than with a bath towel. Do not put the dryer too close to your skin, or use it in the bathroom. Adding a cup of salt to the bath water will also help the stitches to heal.

GETTING BACK INTO SHAPE
Despite losing the combined weight of the baby, the placenta, and the amniotic fluid, you will still be heavier than you were before you became pregnant. You may even find that you have to continue to wear maternity clothes for a short while. As your uterus shrinks during the six

weeks following the birth you will lose more weight, but you will need to watch your diet to regain your pre-pregnancy shape. Try to eat regularly and healthily and don't be tempted, because you're short of time, to snack on foods containing empty calories such as sweets and sodas. If the weight isn't disappearing as fast as you'd like, ask your doctor for advice. Do not attempt any diet now or while breastfeeding – this would just increase stress as your body is trying to regain its equilibrium. Doing exercises will help you get

1 *Waist trimmer: Lie on the floor with your arms away from your side, with your knees bent and feet flat. Pull in your abdominals and, with knees together, roll over to the right. Bring your knees back to the middle and pause.*

2 *Rest briefly, then pull in your abdominals again and roll your knees to the left, then back to the middle and pause. Keep your shoulders flat on the floor as you roll from side to side. Repeat six times and work up to 20.*

1 *Foot exercises: These will help improve your circulation and are especially important if you are confined to bed. Lie with your legs straight and knees together and bend and stretch your feet.*

2 *Flex one foot, pulling the toes up toward you while pointing the other foot away from you. Repeat, alternating the feet. Do this exercise quite briskly for about 30 seconds.*

Post-partum depression

Two or three days after the birth you may suddenly feel very tearful and depressed. This is commonly called the "baby blues," or the milk blues, because it usually coincides with the milk coming into your breasts. These feelings are caused by all the hormonal changes that are going on in your body and should disappear after a few days. If they don't go away, however, you need to talk to your doctor. You may be suffering from post-partum depression

(PPD) which, if left untreated, can go on for several months. Symptoms of PPD include feeling unhappy as well as irritable and exhausted, yet unable to sleep. You may also lose all interest in food, or find yourself eating too much and then feeling guilty afterward. PPD is one of the most common problems following childbirth and it is likely that it is related to the huge hormonal changes that take place at the time of the birth, but it is still unclear as to why it affects some women

so badly but not others. If you think you are suffering from PPD, don't feel ashamed about it and don't ignore the symptoms. You are in need of help and the sooner you ask for it the sooner you will begin to feel better and able to cope with your life again. Post-partum depression is a common condition. Many women are affected by it, and it needs to be treated early on, not just ignored in the hope that eventually it will just go away on its own.

your figure back, get you moving again, and make you feel fitter. Those for strengthening the pelvic floor are among the most important post-partum exercises. The pelvic floor muscles support the bladder, uterus, and rectum, so it is vital that their tone is restored after being stretched during childbirth.

FATIGUE AND RELAXATION

Fatigue goes hand in hand with being a new mother, but you need rest to help your body recover from childbirth. It is tempting to use the baby's sleep times to catch up on chores, but do try to have a nap or proper rest at least once during the day. You and your child are more important than housework, so find ways to cut down the work. Accept offers of help and, if no one volunteers, don't be afraid to ask people.

Another way to cope with fatigue or stress is relaxation, so try using the prenatal relaxation exercises to help you now. For a real treat, ask your partner to give you a massage using a specially formulated oil before you go to sleep. Baths are generally not recommended until after bleeding stops.

HAIR AND NAILS

The condition of your hair is likely to change during this time. It may become more greasy, or the opposite may happen and it will become noticeably drier than before. You may also suffer an increase in hair loss or your hair may seem a lot thicker than it did before you

became pregnant. Whichever condition applies to you, wash your hair
using a mild shampoo and avoid
rubbing or brushing oily hair too
much as this will only stimulate the
sebaceous glands to produce more
oil. Dry hair should be conditioned
after every wash and, if possible,
allowed to dry naturally.

Your nails are made of the same
tissue as your hair, so if you are having problems with one you are likely
to have problems with the other.
These are due to fluctuating hormone levels and as soon as these settle your hair and nails will return to
normal. Meanwhile, include enough
protein and B vitamins in your diet
because these will help improve the
condition of both your hair and nails.

*Left: When bleeding has stopped, a lazy
bath with a few drops of oil, such as
lavender, will help you to relax.*
*Below: A stimulating rub with a loofah
brush or mitt will help remove dead cells
on the skin's surface, and will stimulate
the circulation.*
*Below right: Try using some unscented
soap or a soapless cleansing bar if your
skin is very itchy.*

Above: Eating regularly and healthily will help you to regain your pre-pregnancy shape.

GLOSSARY OF PREGNANCY TERMS

ABORTION
The spontaneous or induced delivery of the fetus before the 28th week.

ABRUPTIO PLACENTAE
Part of the placenta peels away from the wall of the uterus in late pregnancy and often results in bleeding.

ALPHAFETOPROTEIN (AFP)
A protein produced by the fetus that enters the mother's bloodstream. A very high level can indicate neural tube defects of the fetus such as spina bifida, but it can also mean the woman is carrying more than one child.

AMNIOCENTESIS
A small amount of amniotic fluid is taken from the uterus through a needle inserted through the woman's abdomen and tested for chromosomal disorders such as Down's syndrome.

AMNIOTIC FLUID
The fluid surrounding the fetus in the uterus.

AMNIOTIC SAC
The bag of membranes that is filled with amniotic fluid in which the fetus floats during pregnancy.

ANALGESICS
Painkilling drugs which do not cause unconsciousness. The analgesics most commonly used during labor are meperidine hydrochloride (Demerol) and alphaprodine hydrochloride (Nisentil).

ANEMIA
A condition where the level of red corpuscles in the blood are abnormally low, which is treated with iron supplements.

APGAR SCORE
A simple test to assess the baby's condition after birth.

BEARING DOWN
The pushing movement made by the uterus during the second stage of labor.

BIRTH CANAL
See Vagina.

BLASTOCYST
The early stage of the developing embryo when it becomes a cluster of cells.

BRAXTON HICKS CONTRACTIONS
Contractions of the uterus which occur throughout pregnancy, but may not be felt until the last month or so. They feel like a painless, but sometimes uncomfortable, hardening across the stomach.

BREECH PRESENTATION
The position of a baby when he is bottom down rather than head down in the uterus.

CAESARIAN SECTION
Delivery of the baby through a cut in the abdomen and uterine walls.

CERVIX
The neck of the uterus or womb which is sealed with a plug of mucus during pregnancy. During labor, muscular contractions open up the cervix until it is about 4 in wide so that the baby can pass through it into the vagina.

CHLOASMA
Slight discoloration of the skin, usually on the face, which occurs during pregnancy and disappears within weeks of the birth.

CHORIONIC VILLUS SAMPLING
A screening test for genetic handicap which can be done as early as 11 weeks. Cells are taken from the tissue that surrounds the fetus and are then analyzed.

COLOSTRUM
A fluid that the breasts produce during pregnancy and immediately after the birth. It is full of nutrients and contains antibodies which will protect the baby from some infections.

CONCEPTION
The fertilization of the egg by the sperm and its implantation in the wall of the uterus.

CONGENITAL ABNORMALITIES
An abnormality or deformity that exists from birth. It is caused by a damaged gene or the effect of some diseases during pregnancy.

CONTRACTIONS
Regular tightening of the muscles of the uterus as they work to dilate the cervix and push the baby down the birth canal.

CROWNING
The moment when the crown of the baby's head appears in the vagina.

DEMEROL
A drug given during labor for pain relief and relaxation.

DILATION
The gradual opening of the cervix during labor.

DOPPLER
A method of using ultrasound vibrations to listen to the fetal heart.

ECTOPIC PREGNANCY
A pregnancy that develops outside the uterus, usually in the fallopian tube.

EDD
Estimated date of delivery.

EDEMA
Swelling caused by fluid retention.

ELECTIVE INDUCTION
Induction done for convenience rather than for medical reasons.

ELECTRONIC FETAL MONITORING
The continuous monitoring of the fetal heart.

EMBRYO
The name of the developing organism in pregnancy from about the 10th day after fertilization until the 12th week of pregnancy when it becomes known as a fetus.

ENGAGED
The baby's head is engaged when it drops down deep in the pelvic cavity so that the widest part is through the mother's pelvic brim. Another term for this is "lightening." Most babies are born head first and will have engaged before labor begins.

ENGORGEMENT
The breasts become congested with milk if long periods are left between feedings. This results in painful engorgement.

ENTONOX
Gas and oxygen, a short-term analgesic, now rarely used for inhalation during labor.

EPIDURAL
An anaesthetic that is injected into the fluid surrounding the spinal cord at the base of the spine to relieve pain but leave the mother fully conscious.

EPISIOTOMY
A small cut sometimes made in the perineum to enlarge the vagina if there is a risk of tearing when the baby's head is about to be born.

FALLOPIAN TUBES
Two narrow tubes about 4 in long which lead from the ovaries to the uterus.

FETUS
The developing baby from the end of the embryonic stage at about the 12th week of pregnancy, until the date of delivery.

FH
Fetal heart.

FMF
Fetal movement felt.

FOLIC ACID
A form of vitamin B that is important for the healthy development of the embryo. A daily supplement of 0.4mg should be taken before becoming pregnant and then until the 12th week of pregnancy.

FONTANELLES
The soft spots between the unjoined sections of the skull of the baby.

FORCEPS
An instrument sometimes used to assist the baby out of the birth canal.

FOREMILK
The first breast milk the baby gets when he begins to suck which satisfies his thirst before the hind milk comes through.

FUNDUS
The top of the uterus.

GAS AND AIR
See Entonox

GENETIC COUNSELING
Advice on the detection and risk of recurrence of inherited disorders.

GESTATION
The length of time between conception and delivery (usually around 40 weeks).

HEMOGLOBIN (HB)
The pigment that gives blood its red color and contains iron and stores oxygen.

HEMORRHAGE
Excessive bleeding

HEMORRHOIDS
A form of varicose veins around the anus.

HINDMILK
The calorie-rich breast milk that forms the foremilk during feed.

HORMONE
A chemical produced by the body to stimulate organs within the body, particularly those to do with growth and reproduction,

HUMAN CHORIONIC GONADOTROPHIN (HCG)
A hormone produced early in pregnancy by the developing placenta. Its presence in the urine is used to confirm pregnancy.

IMPLANTATION
The embedding of the fertilized egg in the wall of the uterus.

INCOMPETENT CERVIX
A weakened cervix that is unable to hold the fetus in the uterus for the full nine months. Sometimes a cause of late miscarriage or premature birth.

INDUCTION
The process of artificially starting off labor.

INTRAVENOUS DRIP
The infusion of fluids directly into the blood stream through a fine tube into a vein.

JAUNDICE
Neonatal jaundice often occurs in newborn babies because of the inability of the liver to successfully break down an excess of red blood cells.

LABOR
The process of childbirth.

LANUGO
A very fine covering of hair that appears all over the fetus during late pregnancy.

LIE
The position of the fetus in the uterus.

LIGHTENING
See Engaged.

LINEA NIGRA
A line of dark pigmentation that appears down the center of the abdomen on some women during pregnancy.

LOCHIA
Post-partum vaginal discharge

MECONIUM
The green matter passed from the baby's bowels during the first days after birth. Meconium in the amniotic fluid before delivery is usually a sign of fetal distress.

MISCARRIAGE
The loss of a baby before 24 weeks gestation.

MONITOR
Machine or instrument to measure the baby's heartbeat and breathing.

MOLDING
The shaping of the bones of the baby's skull as it passes through the birth canal.

MUCUS
A sticky secretion.

NAD
A medical term often used on medical records meaning "nothing abnormal detected."

NEURAL TUBE DEFECT
Development defect of the brain and/or spinal cord.

OBSTETRICIAN
Medical specialist in pregnancy and childbirth.

OVARY
Female organ responsible for production of sex hormones and eggs (ova).

OVULATION
The production of a ripe egg by the ovary, usually on a monthly basis.

PALPATION
Manual examination of the uterus through the wall of the abdomen.

PELVIC FLOOR
The muscles that support the bladder and the uterus.

PERINATAL
Period from before delivery until seven days after the birth.

PERINEUM
The area between the opening of the vagina and the anus.

PLACENTA
Also known as "afterbirth," this is the fetus's life-support system which is attached to one side of the wall of the uterus and to the baby by means of the umbilical cord. All the fetus's nourishment passes from the mother through the placenta while the fetus's waste products pass out through it.

PREMATURE OR PRETERM
A baby born before the 37th week.

PRE-NATAL
Before birth.

PRESENTATION
The position of the fetus in the uterus before and during the delivery.

PRIMIPARA
A woman who is having her first baby.

PROSTAGLANDIN
A hormone that stimulates the onset of labor contractions.

QUICKENING
The first movements of the fetus in the uterus.

ROOTING
The baby's instinctive searching for the mother's nipple

RUBELLA (GERMAN MEASLES)
A virus that can be dangerous if caught during the first three months of pregnancy.

SHOW
A vaginal discharge of blood-stained mucus that occurs before or during labor

STILLBIRTH
The delivery of a baby who has already died in the uterus after 28 weeks of pregnancy.

STRETCH MARKS
Silvery lines that may appear where the skin has been stretched during pregnancy.

TERM
The end of pregnancy – around 40 weeks from the date of conception.

TERMINATION
An artificially induced abortion before the end of 28th week of pregnancy.

TOXOPLASMOSIS
A parasitic disease spread by cat feces that can cause blindness in a baby.

TRIMESTER
Pregnancy is divided into three trimesters, each making one third of pregnancy.

ULTRASOUND SCAN
A way of screening the fetus in the uterus by bouncing high-frequency sound waves off it which build up a picture.

UMBILICAL CORD
The cord connecting the fetus to the placenta.

UTERUS (WOMB)
The hollow muscular organ in which the fertile egg becomes embedded.

VACUUM EXTRACTOR
An instrument sometimes used to pull the baby out of the vagina.

VAGINA
The birth canal through which the baby makes its way from the uterus.

INDEX

USEFUL ADDRESSES

There is no need to feel alone during pregnancy or in the months after the birth.
The organizations mentioned below are happy to offer help and support to anyone who contacts them.
Remember to enclose an SASE when writing to them.

BIRTHING CHOICES
Academy of Certified Birth Educators,
2001 East Prairie Circle, Suite 1,
Olathe, KS 66062
913-782-5116

American Foundation for Maternal and Child Health,
30 Beekman Place, New York,
NY 10022.
212-759-5510

ASPO/Lamaze,
1840 Wilson Boulevard, Suite 204,
Arlington, VA 22201.

Cesarean/Support, Education and Concern,
22 Forest Road, Framingham, MA
01701.
617-738-6750

Positive Pregnancy and Parenting Fitness,
51 Saltrock Road, Baltic, CT 06330.
203-822-8573

BREASTFEEDING
Human Lactation Center,
666 Sturges Highway, Westport, CT
06880.
203-259-5995

La Leche League International,
P.O. Box 1209, Franklin Park, IL
60131.
708-455-7730

FERTILITY
American Fertility Society,
1209 Montgomery Highway,
Birmingham, AL 35216.
205-978-5000

Vanderbilt University for Fertility and Reproductive Research IVF Program,
D-3200 Medical Center North,
Nashville, TN 37232.

GENERAL HEALTH
American College of Nurse/Midwives,
1522 K. Street NW, Suite 1000,
Washington, DC 20005.
202-289-0171

American College of Obstetricians and Gyneclogists,
409 12th Street SW, Washington,
DC 20037.
202-466-3825

Association of Reproductive Health Professionals,
2401 Pennysylvania Avenue, NW, Suite
350, Washington DC 20037.
202-466-3825

National Women's Health Network,
1325 G Street, NW, LL,
Washington, DC 20005.
202-347-1140

Office on Women's Health,
200 Independence Avenue, SW
Washington, DC 20201.
202-690-7650

GENETIC COUNSELING
Alliance of Genetic Support Groups, 35 Winsconsin Circle, Suite
440, Chevy Chase, MD 20815.
800-336-GENE

National Society for Genetic Counselors,
233 Canterbury Drive, Wallingford,
PA 19086.
215-872-7608

National Network to Prevent Birth Defects,
Box 15309 S.E. Station, Washington,
DC 20003.
202-543-5450

MISCELLANEOUS
International Twins Association,
P.O. Box 77386, Station C, Atlanta,
GA 30357.

Parents without Partners,
8807 Colesville Road, Silver Spring,
MD 20910.

Postpartum Support International
215-295-3994; 805-682-7529
(self-help organization for post-partum
depression)